WHY

IT

HURTS

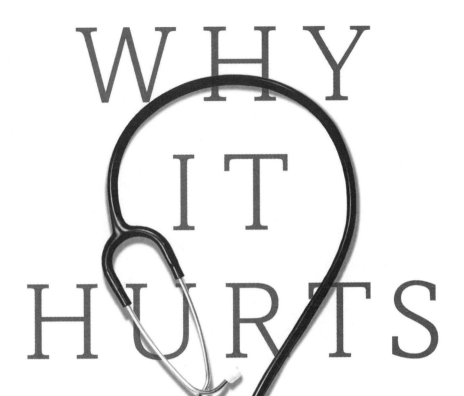

A PHYSICIAN'S

INSIGHTS

ON THE

PURPOSE OF PAIN

D0906364

ANEESH SINGLA, MD

FOR MY PARENTS

CONTENTS

INTRODUCTION

AT SOME POINT IN our lives, we've all wondered if pain is *truly* necessary, and whether modern medicine wouldn't one day simply find a way to turn it off permanently. Maybe you thought about it, after getting that first bee sting in the backyard or after suffering that second-degree burn while "helping" Mom in the kitchen. That searing, thought-scattering sensation shocks us into the present, hurting at the site of the injury and somehow all over at once, leaving us to wonder, *"Why must we feel pain?"*

Pain, in short, is unpleasant. In many ways, it is the polar opposite of everything we enjoy in life, the yin to pleasure's yang. It is also complex and fascinating, an essential element of our experience, as it is indispensable to our overall well-being, as the treasured capacity to feel pleasure. Pain is fundamental to life.

Pain is in another more mundane sense, a colossal problem. Over 116 million Americans suffer from chronic pain, and that pain costs us over $635 billion annually in the U.S. alone.

I have spent over a decade practicing the science—and art—of managing pain as a physician specializing in its treatment.

By sharing my experiences, I hope to shed some light on a difficult and frightening subject. In transforming your perspective on pain—revealing its protective function and life-nurturing purpose—I hope to help you develop resilience, whether you are coping with chronic pain, caring for someone who is, or simply seeking a deeper understanding of a profoundly important subject.

As patients and physicians working together, how aggressively should we treat pain? What is "good" pain versus "bad" pain? When pain is truly unavoidable, how do we make the best of the situation? How do we become better equipped to use our pain as the powerful adaptive tool that it can be?

Although this book is about pain, on a deeper level it is about resilience, healing, and growth. Pain helps reveal the root causes of what ails us. It is a highly developed alarm system the body uses to help us prevent further injury and properly attend to our underlying conditions.

Despite being part of a remarkably sophisticated process, physical pain can be very mysterious when used as a diagnostic tool. Doctors can accurately measure a person's red blood cell count, vitamin D level, or blood glucose level, but to this day we do not have a simple blood test or scan to reliably reveal the source of pain. As healers, doctors face a deductive process combining patient self-reports with clinical findings and the impact of known interventions. Following these diagnostic steps, we do our best to treat the underlying cause. If it is not a "fixable" problem, we aim to relieve the patient's suffering as best we can without causing more harm. It's *always* a delicate balance.

Doctors also encounter physical pain's close relative, psychological pain, which we often label *suffering*. Of course, the mind is intrinsically linked to how we experience all pain. How do we put psychological pain into perspective? This is highly individual. In my experience, psychological pain is even more difficult to understand. Clearly there is a relationship between physical and psychological pain, and yet as a society we place far more emphasis on the former than on the latter, a misconception I also hope to address in this book.

In my own practice as a pain management specialist, I have often wondered about the deeper meaning of pain. This book is the result of that ongoing reflection. In these pages, I recount conversations I've had and situations I've encountered over the years in my work. I attempt to offer a sense of the different ways people experience their pain, think about it, and frame it as part of the larger whole of their existence. While many questions still linger for me, I am certain of one thing: Our beliefs about our pain are crucial to the nature and intensity of our suffering.

A disclaimer: while writing this book, I've worked hard to reflect on my experiences, as objectively as possible. I have incorporated the latest research, notes from observers, and, above all, feedback from patients. But pain is as subjective as anything in the human experience. So keep in mind that everything you read here is interpreted through my own beliefs, preferences, and prejudices as a pain specialist and as a person. Your mileage, as they say, will vary.

The process of writing this book has been therapeutic for me. It has allowed me to dwell on and deeply consider aspects of pain that often go overlooked in the day-to-day operation of a busy pain management practice. It has given me the opportunity to step outside my primary field of expertise, delving into the literature of psychology, business, military history, mythology, and more in the search for collective wisdom and new perspectives on the subject at hand.

In my work as a pain physician, I follow the path set by my patients' physical and psychological symptoms to guide me to the root cause of their pain. Often, conversations with my patients lead me toward a better understanding of the complexities of pain. Their questions have inspired me to go on this quest for answers that might help them better understand their experience.

I make no claims of completeness. I've only scratched the surface in these pages and I am certain you will leave this book with more questions about pain than answers. However, I have done my best to patiently assemble some of the pieces of the puzzle together. Perhaps reading this book will help you begin to form a picture of the completed puzzle in your mind. You may also gain some insight into painful experiences in your own life.

One final note: in the following chapters, I share stories from real patients. I hope these will resonate with you, not just in terms of the pain they experienced but also in the joy, recovery, and wisdom they display. I have changed patient names and identifying details but the essential elements of every case study are true.

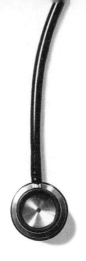

CHAPTER 1

WHAT IS PAIN?

> Think of pain as a speech your body is delivering
> about a subject of vital importance to you.
>
> —PAUL BRAND, *The Gift of Pain: Why We Hurt &*
> *What We Can Do About It*

ONE SUNDAY AFTERNOON WHILE cleaning out my garage, I noticed some bottles of beer that needed to be moved to the refrigerator. I picked them up and, as I turned to open the fridge door, one slipped out of the carton and smashed on the concrete floor behind me. The pressurized liquid sounded like an explosion. Shards of glass lay scattered across the garage floor. When I knelt down to sweep them up, I noticed a twinge in my left leg. Upon examining my calf, I discovered a two-inch-long gash, but I hadn't felt anything at the time of the injury. The explosive sound had startled me so much, it had completely distracted me from the experience of the injury.

Physical pain is a universal experience. (There are certain people who do not feel pain, as we will discuss in Chapter 2, but they are extraordinarily rare exceptions.) While the sensation is unpleasant—at best—it serves a vital function by teaching us how to adapt to our surroundings.

For example, when we are young, we learn that we experience pain when we touch something sharp. Thus, we learn to avoid sharp objects to avoid further damaging our bodies. Pain, in short, is an adaptive and protective sensation.

TYPES OF PHYSICAL PAIN

The body uses physical pain to get our attention when something is amiss. Someone's jaw hurts; the dentist discovers an infected tooth and pulls it. Someone's abdomen hurts; the family doctor diagnoses appendicitis and orders an emergency appendectomy. These pains are *acute*. Acute pain develops immediately after an injury or another distinct event. By contrast, *chronic* pain develops over time and generally lasts for months or longer.

Acute and chronic physical pain can be further classified as *inflammatory, nociceptive,* or *pathological*. Rheumatoid arthritis and osteoarthritis are two familiar kinds of inflammatory pain. Inflammation occurs when our immune system responds to an injury by sending an army of infection-fighting cells to destroy invaders in our bodies. This response results in warmth, swelling, and hypersensitivity, along with pain. In the case of an autoimmune disease like rheumatoid arthritis, the body mounts an immune response to harmless tissue that is misinterpreted as dangerous. This results in infection-fighting cells, which produce antibodies, to attack the cushioning and shock-absorbing cartilage in our joints.

"Doc," one patient with arthritis said, "my hip feels like I have a constant toothache." His pain was chronic and inflammatory.

Nociceptive pain results from physical trauma such as a skin laceration or a burn from a hot stove. It's a response by the nervous system to a physical event that damages our body. This is generally a sharp, stabbing, or cutting sensation in the area of the injury, depending on the type of damage inflicted. Acute, nociceptive pain is what I experienced when I bent down to clean the garage floor and discovered the gash on my calf.

Pathological, sometimes called neuropathic, pain has no adaptive purpose. In fact, it is often referred to as *maladaptive* pain because it provides no specific protective function. From an evolutionary perspective, it does not confer a survival advantage. Typically, this type of pain is due to nerve injury or nervous system dysfunction. Depending on the type of nerve involved, a patient suffering from pathological pain might feel a burning, stabbing, or electrical sensation with no injury to account for it. As you can imagine, this kind of pain presents unique challenges for diagnosis and management because it is more difficult to identify its underlying cause.

Unlike neuropathic pain, inflammatory and nociceptive pains are considered to be *adaptive*. Think of a smoke detector. Working properly, it sounds an alarm whenever there is enough smoke in the air to indicate a fire. Thus, it serves a vital adaptive function: alerting you to evacuate before your house burns down. Adaptive pain is the body's smoke detector. It signals an alarm—a pain sensation—whenever pain receptors are triggered by damage to your cells. It's the body's way of saying, "Take your hand off that stove before the burn gets any worse." That is a classic example of nociceptive pain.

When you do get a burn, on your finger for instance, the pain you feel for days afterward is inflammatory. This is the pain from the inflammation response at the site of the healing tissue. The body's smoke alarm is still serving its purpose by alerting you that the cells are busy healing injured tissue. Even though it's annoying, the inflammatory pain is there for a very good reason: to tell you that your finger is not ready for the next task at hand. Achy, tired joints and muscles while fighting off the flu are another example of adaptive inflammatory pain. In this case, the pain suggests you rest and let the body fight off the virus.

Of course, smoke detectors aren't always right. Sometimes, they go off when there's a bit of smoke but no danger of a house fire. For example, I recently overdid it searing some salmon for dinner. Off goes the ear-piercing smoke alarm, and up the ladder I go to wave the smoke away. In the body, this kind of false alarm is known as pathological pain and, unfortunately, waving a towel around it isn't going to help.

Pathological pain is a kind of hurt that occurs when an acute injury hasn't occurred, a maladaptive pain. For example, people with trigeminal neuralgia, also known as tic douloureux, experience severe jaw pain. There is nothing physically wrong with the jaw, but the pain alarm sounds loudly and ceaselessly, without serving any adaptive or protective purpose.

When someone presents with any type of physical pain, one of the first steps in evaluating the problem is to ask a series of diagnostic questions: Where does it hurt? Does it radiate?

Would you describe it as sharp or dull? Shooting? Can you give a number to your pain, with zero being no pain and ten being the worst pain imaginable?

Doctors may order a barrage of tests: X-rays, MRIs, blood work, and so on. They then try to piece it all together to form a diagnosis. When a cause is detected, the patient is either sent to a specialist (e.g., a urologist to treat a kidney stone) or treated on the spot (e.g., with antibiotics for a urinary tract infection). In cases of pathological pain, however, test results may show nothing abnormal. Such perplexing cases usually require the intervention of a pain specialist like me.

Beyond inflammatory, nociceptive, and pathological pain, there is the realm of psychological pain. Both physical and psychological pains require a diagnostic workup to get to the underlying cause. There are parallels in the diagnostic processes of a psychologist or psychiatrist: "I see you are anxious and depressed. Can you describe the sensation of your anxiety? Do you know what kinds of situations trigger your depression?"

Anxiety, with or without pain, can be adaptive. For example, if you're worried about an upcoming test, your anxiety may push you to study. As you firm up your knowledge of the test material, your anxiety should fade. Anxiety can also be maladaptive. If you suffer from an anxiety disorder like agoraphobia, the irrational fear of open spaces, it can prevent you from even holding a job that requires leaving the house. This would require proper psychiatric treatment to regain normal function. (We discuss psychological pain further in Chapter 3.)

Pain is unpleasant; it needs to be. If it weren't, we'd ignore it. Think about that time the low-fuel indicator came on in your car and you kept driving. (How did you like that walk to the gas station in 90-degree heat?) Pain is painful precisely because it needs to jolt us into action.

* * *

Let's return to the garage on that Sunday afternoon when I was moving beer into the fridge. The gash on my leg was starting to throb and burn. I tried unsuccessfully to bandage it; it was bleeding too profusely. It looked like stitches would be necessary, given the size and depth of the laceration. Reluctantly, I told my wife and daughter that I'd be missing the family trip to the neighborhood pool. Instead, I hopped in the car, saw and ignored the low fuel indicator, and drove to the nearest emergency room.

"Insurance card and ID please?"

After filling out the forms, feeling a bit sheepish considering how minor my injury was compared to those I saw around me, I buried myself in an outdated magazine and tried to get comfortable.

Physical pain helps us survive life-threatening situations by activating our fight-or-flight system. When it detects danger, our body releases adrenaline and other chemicals to help us run faster, jump higher, and focus more clearly on the threat at hand—our survival depends on it. So when the smoke detector is going off for no reason, as it does with maladaptive pain, it can't simply be ignored. Chronic pain gnaws away at you because millions of years of evolution have designed pain to command your attention. This wears you down quickly and adds a component of psychological pain to the picture.

As a pain specialist, I seek to diagnose the root cause of adaptive or maladaptive pain from a constellation of symptoms. I order laboratory tests, perform clinical examinations, and use every other tool at my disposal to confirm or refute a list of possible diagnoses until I've narrowed it down to the most likely culprit. While there's no doubt that pain exists when a patient reports it, I have to keep the subjective experience of the patient in mind as I look for a possible physical source.

When the source of pain is hard to identify, people become desperate. This is natural, but their despair can actually amplify their pain sensation. No matter how unpleasant the pain, it isn't wise to seek to turn the sensation off entirely. One of my patients, Mark, suffered from severe complex regional pain syndrome (CRPS), a painful condition of sharp, shooting, burning pain in the arms or legs. This syndrome can occur after an injury. The nerves get stuck in a circular feedback loop: The pain produces inflammation, then the inflammation produces more pain. The sympathetic nervous system, which controls a person's fight-or-flight response, facilitates something we call *wind-up*. The pain in the affected area worsens and worsens.

To understand this phenomenon, think of the volume control on your stereo. You turn the knob up and the "volume" of the music is increased—and each note is amplified many times higher. In the nervous system, the pain signal is progressively turned up many times higher through wind-up. In a pain circular feedback loop, the nervous system continues to wind up, so the intensity of the pain increases over time.

By the time of his appointment, Mark was experiencing extraordinarily severe pain in his leg.

"Can't you just cut the leg off?" Mark asked. That question should give you some sense of the desperation chronic pain patients experience.

Mark isn't my only patient with nerve damage to have asked about surgically removing a limb. I empathize deeply with anyone whose suffering has reached the point where amputation seems like a feasible alternative. Unfortunately, as I tell my patients, severing the limb in question would actually make the pain much worse due to *central sensitization*, a phenomenon where pain sensation actually increases due to the nervous system's sensitivity going into overdrive. Think of central sensitization as the end result of wind-up. It is the new set point for your nervous system. Going back to the volume control example, your centrally sensitized nervous system is now where the volume has been turned up on your body's stereo.

To give you a sense of how bad pathological pain can feel, here's an excerpt from *The Story of Pain* by Joanna Bourke, quoting physician Valentine Mott:

I have seen the most heroic and stout-hearted men shed tears like a child, when enduring the agony of neuralgia. As in a powerful engine when the director turns some little key, and the monster is at once aroused, and plunges along the pathway, screaming and breathing forth flames in the majesty of his power, so the hero of a hundred battles, if perchance a filament of nerve is compressed, is seized with spasms, and struggles to escape the unendurable agony.

Mott puts it more poetically than I ever could, but his description resonates with what I've witnessed as a pain specialist.

PAIN AND THE WITHDRAWAL REFLEX

But pointless suffering is only part of the picture. Pain is essential in helping us process and interpret our environment. It is no understatement to say that pain is vital to life and to our survival as a species.

We have many reflexes that help us adapt and survive, and pain plays a part in many of them. The withdrawal reflex, triggered by pain, drives us to unconsciously pull back from potentially damaging situations. When our eyes dry out or come in contact with dust or a foreign object, the trigeminal nerve detects this discomfort and signals our brain, which in turn tells the facial nerve to tell our eyelid to blink. This blink reflex helps lubricate the eye to keep the cornea from drying out.

You can override the blink reflex, but it's uncomfortable. Think of your last staring contest, or of the effort of keeping your eyes open during the flash of a family photo. Both of these are examples of how you can modulate the blink reflex by focusing on and inhibiting it. Overriding the blink reflex for too long is not only uncomfortable, but it can also result in damage to your eye. To an extent, the same is true for the adaptive side of pain. We can modulate its actions and severity, but in the end we need it to survive.

Other common reflexes include the cough reflex, which might be triggered when food goes down your windpipe, and the itch reflex, which alerts you to scratch when mosquitoes are making unsanctioned withdrawals from your blood supply.

These involuntary actions are common, protective responses that are usually adaptive. While they each have the potential to become maladaptive in certain situations—a chronic cough after a cold, the ceaseless itch of an allergic reaction—we have to keep their protective qualities in mind as we cope with them. Pain is no different.

One example of the many subtle ways pain protects you below the level of conscious thought happens when we run. If you pay attention during a run, you'll notice yourself automatically making adjustments to your gait as you go. This is the pain reflex warning you whenever an area of your body experiences too much repetitive stress so you can adjust your stride before lasting damage—a torn ligament, a sprained ankle—occurs.

It's not quite as immediate a reaction as the blink reflex, but it still involves input that travels from an extremity through your spinal cord to your brain, where it is processed. In response, your brain sends instructions to compensate. While it's likely that you process this information subconsciously, the fact remains that pain made you change your behavior. If you couldn't feel that pain, you'd risk getting a blister, a stress fracture, or worse. Pain provides your brain with constant feedback for adjustment, both consciously and subconsciously, every minute of the day.

In *A New Earth: Awakening to Your Life's Purpose*, Eckhart Tolle writes, "The body operates by an intelligence that we don't fully understand." I believe we can learn to recognize and appreciate the intelligence and wisdom of the human body when it comes to pain. We have evolved with the spirit of survival as our most paramount goal; pain facilitates that survival.

If we do not see pain's value, I would argue that we threaten our own survival.

PAIN AS A TOOL FOR GROWTH

Humans thrive on competition in sports, academics, business, the arts, and every other arena. Through both winning and losing, we learn, better ourselves, and set benchmarks for future growth. We compete against others and we compete with ourselves, pushing through that extra repetition at the gym or trimming five seconds off our three-mile run. Pain is essential in honing our competitive edge. It tells us how far we can push and when to back off. When you feel the burn of lactic acid (inflammatory pain) during the last mile of your run or the last set of your workout, you know you are close to your physical limit. That sensation tells you that you can push just a little bit more before you rest in order to maximize the benefit of your training session. When you push yourself to the threshold of discomfort, your muscles tear microscopically. When you rest, they rebuild stronger than before. Pain is essential to this growth process.

The Golgi tendon organ is the sensory receptor that helps us know our limits when we stretch our bodies. Without it to warn us, we would extend our muscles beyond their limits, tearing them and even damaging our joints. Pain regulates both the stretch and the contraction, keeping us safely between both extremes. In order to see the benefits of stretching after a workout, you have to gently push against the limit set by pain. As Benjamin Franklin wrote in his classic essay, *The Way to Wealth*:

So what signifies wishing and hoping for better times? We may make these times better, if we bestir ourselves. Industry need not wish, and he that lives upon hopes will die fasting. There are no gains without pains.

Growth and gains come at a price through pain. The phrase "no pain, no gain" appears in many contexts, but above all in the realm of fitness.

In her book *Unbroken* about World War II prisoner of war (POW) Louis Zamperini, Laura Hillenbrand illustrates the remarkable growth that can accompany a willingness to embrace discomfort. Zamperini was born in America to Italian immigrants. As a boy, he was bullied and mocked for his English, so his father taught him how to box. Training in the ring with his dad involved a lot of discomfort and pain, but Zamperini wanted the bullying to stop, so he pushed through it and eventually began to defend himself successfully.

Zamperini's older brother, Pete, encouraged Louis to start running track. To keep pace, Pete would run behind him and hit him with a switch if he slowed down. Pretty soon, Zamperini was breaking records. A naturally gifted runner, he went on to compete in the 1936 Olympics.

In 1938, Zamperini competed in the mile while at USC. Other runners singled out the Olympian in their midst for abuse, spiking him with the sharp edges of their shoes to hurt him and slow him down. Determined, Zamperini pushed through the pain to set a new record for the national collegiate mile: 4 minutes, 8 seconds.

Without pain or the fear of more pain driving him, Zamperini would never have achieved his amazing potential. Without achieving that potential, he never would have survived the challenges to come.

In 1941, Zamperini joined the Air Force to fight in the Second World War. His plane was shot down over the Pacific and he was captured by the Japanese after a long and arduous 47 days at sea in a raft. Near starvation, Zamperini was put into a POW camp, where he was beaten and tortured. At one point, he was forced to hold a steel beam over his head. Though weakened and pushed to his physical limits, he defied his captors by not succumbing to the pain.

After the war, Zamperini returned home, suffering from nightmares and what we might today call post-traumatic stress disorder (PTSD). He became an alcoholic, descending deeper and deeper into psychological pain. Eventually, however, Zamperini overcame the psychological trauma and alcoholism through a spiritual transformation. He became a Christian evangelist, forgiving his captors. Some of them even converted to Christianity after being embraced by their former prisoner. In a way, Zamperini's remarkable resilience delivered a hopeful lesson to others about easing their own pain.

Pain is a metaphor that we can all relate to- -it is especially valuable when it helps us remember a significant event, such as childbirth. Pain brings home the poignancy of the key events of our lives. Without pain, we would not appreciate the limits of our bodies and rally behind those who seek to test those limits. People facing physical challenges could not know their body's limits without pain. By enduring the discomfort, victory is sweeter. We can all learn to better ourselves, through the embodied wisdom in pain, to become more resilient when faced with life's challenges.

PUSHING THROUGH THE PAIN

Medicine is an art as well as a science. When it comes to the care of patients with maladaptive pain, there is a great deal of art involved because the science of pain is still very much in its infancy. Pain is both crucial and complex, nothing to be treated lightly. We must embrace what it tells us, because avoiding it completely simply isn't an option.

"So what do I do when I get the pain?" asks Bob, a patient with spinal stenosis. "Stop and sit down until it gets better, or push through it?" Spinal stenosis is a narrowing of a region of the spine. In the lumbar spine region, it causes lower back pain and numbness in the legs when you stand or walk too long. Sit down, and the pain usually resolves within minutes.

"This is anything but a no-pain, no-gain situation," I tell him. "Let your pain tell you when to rest and when it's okay to get up again."

Physicians are notorious for tolerating discomfort many others would not as they undergo the rigorous training and punishing hours of medical school, residencies, and beyond. How are *we* supposed to know when a patient is on the right path when we are treating their pain? Do we draw an arbitrary line somewhere in the sand?

In *When Breath Becomes Air*, Paul Kalanithi relates the pain he experienced from stage IV lung cancer, and how he pushed through that pain to complete his rigorous neurosurgical training at Stanford.

Though he was rapidly coming face to face with his own mortality, his desire to complete the path he was on was stronger than the pain, simple as that. Kalanithi's book is a beautiful account of pain faced and overcome. Pain makes us present to our lives in a way that would not be possible without it. One passage illustrates the remarkable relationship between pain, suffering, and meaning:

> A bevy of new pain medications was prescribed. As I hobbled out of the hospital, I wondered how, just six days ago, I had spent nearly thirty-six straight hours in the operating room...and even so, I had suffered excruciating pain... Yes, I thought, and therein was the paradox: like a runner crossing the finish line only to collapse, without that duty to care for the ill pushing me forward, I became an invalid.

Kalanithi's mission to become a healer made it possible for him to accomplish anything in the face of extraordinary pain.

THE HUMAN RESPONSE TO PAIN

Humans remember painful things like nothing else. From hazing rituals and other rites of passage, to childbirth and injuries or illnesses, events involving intense pain are etched into our memories. Depending on the story we tell ourselves about our suffering, they are often remembered as transformative events, experiences that turned us into who we have become.

As I sat in the emergency room waiting for someone to stitch up my leg, I wondered what I could have done differently: pick up the bottles one by one? Take my time instead of rushing? Wear pants instead of shorts? A dozen thoughts went through my mind. It's human nature to imagine alternatives when an accident occurs. We seek the lesson in the pain when it isn't obvious.

Some patients are shocked when I tell them there is an upside to pain, but this mindset is crucial to our survival. The downside of having no pain is far worse, as we will see in Chapter 2. In Kelly McGonigal's book *The Upside of Stress,* she makes a similar argument about stress. Using stress as a positive or adaptive force that pushes you to overcome the challenge ahead is far healthier in the long run than trying to avoid stress. We feel stress because what we're doing matters to us.

There is something similar to be said about pain. In fact, stress can exacerbate pain and vice versa, but with the right mindset you can use these feelings as a catalyst to energize yourself, when you turn your thoughts towards the task at hand.

The concept of learning from our mistakes is in many ways about learning from our pain. Mistakes are painful—physically as well as psychologically—but we learn from them and use them to better ourselves. Along this journey of trying to better understand pain, I have come to believe that pain is a rich and vital source of learning.

* * *

Eventually, I was brought to an exam room and asked to sit on a gurney. The familiar sterile environment was accompanied by the smell of alcohol and polished steel. Everything about it said *hospital.* The physician's assistant greeted me in a no-nonsense manner.

"I'm going to numb you up, wash out the wound, and sew you up," she said. "Okay?" I lay down on my side. As she worked, I prided myself for not complaining about the pain or showing any outward signs of discomfort. It struck me as funny how strongly conditioned we are not to show pain in modern society, despite the fact that this desire to cry out is adaptive, intended to let others know we need help.

"When was your last tetanus shot?"

"I can't remember." I said, embarrassed. So she gave me another one, just in case. Ouch.

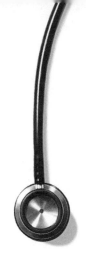

CHAPTER 2

A BLESSING IN DISGUISE

> If you want to make peace with your enemy, you have
> to work with your enemy. Then he becomes your partner.
>
> —NELSON MANDELA

BEFORE THE DISCOVERY OF surgical anesthesia in the mid-1800s, patients were forced to endure the pain of surgery while awake. This must have been a horrifying experience. In her journals, the 19th-century English novelist and playwright Frances Burney recounted the experience of undergoing breast surgery to remove a mass:

> When the dreadful steel was plunged into the breast—cutting through veins—arteries—flesh—nerves—I needed no injunctions not to restrain my cries. I began a scream that lasted unintermittingly during the whole time of the incision—& I almost marvel that it rings not in my Ears still!

Before anesthesia, the merit of a surgeon came down to his speed; this was paramount due to the immense pain patients were experiencing. The need to decrease pain so that surgeons could operate more precisely led to the discovery of surgical anesthesia. Anesthesia allowed surgeons to perform longer, more complex surgical procedures while sparing patients the excruciating pain of their work.

Before the discovery of anesthesia, even the most intense pain was simply accepted as a part of life. Those who suffered turned to religion for solace. It's no coincidence that Karl Marx called religion "the opiate of the masses." C.S. Lewis once wrote that "all great religions were first preached, and long practiced, in a world without chloroform."

In earlier times, pain and disease were thought to be sent from God as punishment for sins and as an opportunity to seek redemption. Throughout the Middle Ages, pain was thought to provide spiritual purification. In Europe and America as late as the 18th century, physicians were often members of the clergy.

Early in the 19th century, a shift in thinking occurred. It began a humanitarian ideology that saw pain as something that should be avoided. Some philosophers began to argue that pain and suffering were fundamentally unnecessary.

In drafting the Declaration of Independence, Thomas Jefferson wrote that we all have a right to "life, liberty, and the pursuit of happiness." This became a part of the ideological bedrock of the United States of America. If Americans had a right to pursue happiness, presumably this included the right to avoid pain.

Nineteenth-century scientific advances were paralleled by increasingly secular attitudes toward pain. There was a growing belief that suffering could be avoided and that it was truly unnecessary. As doctors used the scientific method to relieve ailments, people grew more reliant on science and less dependent on religion as the only available salve for pain and suffering. Despite advancing in other ways, the field of medicine was still years away from developing anesthesia.

Without anesthesia, pain put a major limit on the advancement of medical science. When a surgeon attempted a surgical cure for an illness or affliction, a patient was forced to endure the torture of an operation. There was simply no way around the pain. Some physicians tried using alcohol as a sedative to dull pain. Others asked patients to bite a bullet or use other, similar techniques to distract them from the pain. None of these measures effectively prevented much suffering. At the very least, this new, humanitarian view towards pain and the concomitant belief in the power of science to solve problems drove the search for a safe and effective anesthetic.

In 1846, William T. G. Morton, an American dentist, tried using ether, a gas, to put a patient under before performing a tooth extraction. When his patient awoke after the bloody procedure, he reported having experienced no pain. Morton went on to give the first successful demonstration of general anesthesia at Massachusetts General Hospital[1], putting a patient under with ether while surgeon John Collins Warren removed a tumor.

---

1   Harvard Medical School has three primary teaching hospitals: Massachusetts General Hospital (sometimes referred to simply as "Mass General"), Brigham and Women's Hospital, and Beth Israel Deaconess Hospital.

Warren wrote about the landmark surgery:

> The patient being prepared for the operation, the apparatus was applied to his mouth by Dr. Morton for about three minutes, at the end of which time he sank into a state of insensibility. I immediately made an incision about three inches long through the skin of the neck and began a dissection among important nerves and blood vessels without any expression of pain on the part of the patient... Being asked immediately afterward whether he had suffered much, he said that he had felt as if his neck had been scratched; but subsequently, when inquired of by me, his statement was, that he did not experience pain at the time....

Surgical anesthesia led directly to improved medical care. Now surgeons could focus on the complex operation at hand, taking the much-needed time to perform their work correctly.

Over the years, refinements brought surgical anesthesia to even higher levels. When I began my anesthesiology residency training in 2001, I marveled at the power of surgical anesthesia to quickly and completely shield a patient from the pain of surgery and then to bring them back to full consciousness with no apparent ill effects. The interesting thing is that we still don't really know how anesthesia works to accomplish this, despite its universal use.

A surgeon, frustrated that few of his procedures went exactly as he had planned, turned to me in the operating room.

"Anesthesia is like magic," he said. "It always works!"

Anesthesia forever changed society's attitude on pain and

suffering. It also gave surgeons the confidence that they could now tackle many previously inoperable conditions.

Regional, as opposed to general, anesthesia makes one part of the body numb while the patient is still awake. It gives expectant mothers the option of experiencing little to no pain during childbirth. During my residency, I spent some time on the obstetrics ward. It was immensely gratifying to find a woman in agony from painful contractions and, with the insertion of an epidural, offer her immediate and almost complete relief from that pain. It was like a switch was flipped. Thanks to the invention of regional anesthesia techniques, childbirth pain can be seen as something that may simply be avoided as opposed to something intrinsic to the experience of motherhood.

Both general and regional anesthesia represent tremendous medical advances. Pain management has been a key function of all physicians but, in retrospect, it seems only natural that anesthesiologists would gravitate toward it. After all, the anesthesiologist's expertise lies in managing pain before, during, and after surgery. Why not adapt these powerful techniques for patients suffering with pain outside of the operating room?

That said, when I actually worked at a chronic pain clinic, I became acutely aware of how unsuccessful we were as a specialty field at helping so many sufferers.

If you're reading this book, you probably know that chronic pain is an enormous problem, but you may not realize quite how enormous. Once you account for indirect costs like lost workdays, we spend $635 *billion a year* on chronic pain in the United States alone. Health care represents about 18 percent of our GDP, or about $3 trillion a year. Hard as it is to believe, chronic pain represents the equivalent of one out of every five dollars spent on the *entire* U.S. health care system per year.

I knew we had long ago found effective ways to manage surgical pain. I also knew chronic pain was a colossal source of suffering and a tremendous economic burden. So why, I wondered, hadn't we figured out how to translate all of our scientific understanding of surgical pain into advancing the treatment of chronic, and sometimes even acute, pain?

Teeming with enthusiasm to seek better therapies for pain, I pursued pain management as a subspecialty. I wanted to make an impact where one was so desperately needed. After all, what greater contribution could a healer make than to conquer pain and suffering? All doctors manage their patients' pain in some way, whether after surgical procedure or an ankle sprain, but this was a chance to really fix pain for good. How could I resist?

So I packed my bags and set off to do a fellowship at Brigham and Women's Hospital in Boston. I didn't need to pack much, as it was just across town from where I finished my residency, Massachusetts General Hospital, but the institutional cultures couldn't have been more different.

As I began my career in pain management, I wanted nothing more than to ease the suffering of my patients, and I became more and more frustrated as I realized that I could not do this in every instance. As an anesthesiologist, I could elegantly render patients unconscious so that surgeons could carefully remove a tumor or repair a torn ligament. I could rest assured that as long as I did my job properly, my patients were comfortable.

As a practicing pain specialist, I could only seek to reduce pain to a certain extent; my patients still had to function in the world. But couldn't we just isolate pain? Couldn't we remove pain entirely from our sensory experience while keeping the rest of the body awake and mindful of the environment?

THE TRAGEDY OF LIFE WITHOUT PAIN

Shortly after becoming a pain specialist, I learned of a rare condition that renders a person completely unable to experience pain. Patients with congenital insensitivity to pain (CIP) are normal in every way except for their inability to feel pain, but their syndrome has a severe impact on their lives. The following case appeared in the *Journal of Orthopedic Surgery*:

In March 2010, a 7-month-old boy presented with a 4-day history of increasing swelling of the elbow, pseudo-paralysis of the right upper limb, and high fever. The child appeared to be toxic. The sensation of pain was less than expected. Multiple ulcers were noted over both hands and feet and tongue. Pain perception appeared to be completely absent, which the parents stated had been present since birth. The parents also stated the child frequently had self-inflicted wounds over the hands, feet, and tongue. Injections into the skin to test for a response produced no pain. The right elbow was found to be infected, and the patient was taken to the operating room where about 20 ml of infected pus was drained, and complete separation and dislocation of the joint were seen. The child was placed on antibiotics for four weeks. Unfortunately, the damage and erosion to the joint were so severe, the joint was permanently damaged and showed evidence of chronic lingering infection of the bone, called osteomyelitis.

This child suffered from CIP, a genetic disease occurring in roughly 1 out of every 25,000 people. Children afflicted with it have a short life expectancy because, without pain, they have little to no ability to avoid trauma from accidents. Without the ability to use pain as a protective reflex, they can't reliably avoid the harmful things in their environment. In short, these individuals have no ability to adapt to their environment. Parents of children with CIP cannot trust that a child will cry to indicate that something is wrong and this makes it difficult for them to remedy injuries or illness.

As I learned more about the impact of CIP and other conditions that affect our sensitivity to pain, I began to realize that pain provides a critical survival advantage. When we're caught in its grasp, it can be incredibly difficult to see it in this positive light, but my experience has shown me that pain is actually one of our greatest allies.

I have tried using the metaphor of gravity to help people put pain into perspective. Gravity, like pain, is simply a part of life. It's not going anywhere. Like pain, gravity can shape, challenge, and direct you.

While most people don't think very much about the earth's gravitational force, it affects everything on the planet. For example, it works against a child learning to ride a bike, who must fight to stay balanced or risk scraping a knee. It can be fun to imagine all the things that might be possible if gravity weren't as strong: effortlessly slam-dunking basketballs, gracefully floating through the air. In reality, a gravity-free world would be quite harmful. Without the constant pull of gravity on their bodies, astronauts' muscles and bones atrophy despite the rigorous exercise routines they maintain in orbit. In fact, months in space with little to no gravity result in bones becoming brittle and osteoporotic.

Like gravity, pain helps us. Even though pain is certainly an unpleasant feeling that we have to experience, it would be far more dangerous not to be able to experience it.

Patrick Wall, a pioneer in the field of pain, commented on CIP:

> Let us pause here to consider the fact that, very, very rarely, children are born who grow up with no sensation of pain. [They] have been the subject of intense study because they are so fascinating and test all our ideas about the meaning and usefulness of our normal ability to perceive pain.

In an interview with Wall, a Canadian student at McGill University with CIP reported a strong pinch felt merely like a "strong pressure." Wall continued:

> All her other body sensations—touch, pressure, warm, cold, and movement—appeared completely normal. How had she grown up without the massive protection supposedly provided by the withdrawal reflex? She had continuous monitoring by her doctor father, mother, and siblings, who were all aware of her problem. Gross damage such as a cut, burn, or fracture does not need pain to be rapidly detected by the victim. Appendicitis had been diagnosed in her by the signs of fever, inflammation, and gut motility, even though she had no pain. Unusual accidents do occur

in such people in novel situations. For example, as a child in the deep Canadian winter, she climbed up to look out of the window and knelt on a hot radiator. One could still see the line scars on her knees as an adult.

The Canadian student died at the age of 22 from osteomyelitis, the same bone infection contracted by the infant described in the *Journal of Orthopedic Surgery*. Why? Remember what I said earlier about the constant presence of low-level discomfort in our lives, how even as we jog, our stride adjusts to give breaks to parts of the body taking more than normal stress, so they can recover?

Whenever the student was injured in a minor way, this automatic recovery phase did not occur. The surfaces of her joints and ligaments were never given the time to fully recover from stress. This left them in a perpetually weakened state, ill-equipped to face future trivial injuries.

Counterintuitively, severe injuries such as fractures do not have such severe consequences for CIP sufferers. When a limb is severely damaged, it is simply put in a cast and held stationary until the healing is complete. Repetitive minor injuries, on the other hand, demolish the joints of those with CIP over time, particularly the ankles, knees, and wrists. The dead and damaged tissue in the joints then becomes a haven where bacteria can flourish, eating their way through the bone and into the marrow. This explosive invasion, osteomyelitis, is still extremely difficult to treat, even with antibiotics, because the medicine cannot easily penetrate this deeply into the body.

Learning about CIP brought me back to my work in

anesthesiology. While under anesthesia, patients have to be cared for with vigilance. Nerve injury can occur if, for example, the patient's body moves into the wrong position. Even when we're asleep at home, our bodies feel pain and will adjust to anatomically comfortable positions. Under anesthesia, it falls on the anesthesiologist to vigilantly guard the patient while pain is turned off. Life without pain subjects you to the same need for constant attention.

Golnar Jahanmir, a pediatric dentist at Children's Hospital in Washington, D.C., works with patients with CIP. In some cases, she and her colleagues have had to remove teeth because a child was continuously biting and producing skin erosions in the mouth. For some children with CIP, what should be pain is actually felt as a tingling that actually drives them to physically harm themselves because they find the sensation stimulating. This brings me back to my childhood. When I'd have a numb lip after a dental procedure, all I wanted to do was to keep biting it. Thankfully for me, that numbness was only temporary.

CIP isn't the only way our capacity for pain can be lost. Diabetes, a chronic inability to correctly regulate blood sugar, can damage nerves when blood sugar levels are too high for too long. This nerve damage, called neuropathy, can cause patients to lose sensation in their feet and ankles. As with CIP, diabetic neuropathy makes the feet vulnerable to constant, repetitive stress due to walking or running. Because of the patient's inability to sense the injury, ulcers can eventually occur. Decreased blood flow, also due to diabetes, combined with additional, unremitting pressure on the ulcer can result in infection. By the time these infections are detected, there is often erosion into the bones of the feet, culminating in osteomyelitis. This can result in the loss of the limb or the spread of the infection to other parts of the body.

Another threat to our protective pain response is leprosy. For most of human history, people believed that the disease of leprosy, widespread enough to be mentioned multiple times in the Bible, caused the body's extremities to rot and fall off. But, as first discovered by the English physician Paul Brand, leprosy's true effcct is to damage the nerves that transmit pain.

After completing extensive work with leprosy patients in India, Brand noticed how patients with the disease would constantly injure themselves without realizing it, resulting in skin ulcers and trauma. One experience at the leprosarium opened his eyes to the effects of the disease, as he later related in his book, *The Gift of Pain*:

> A woman...was roasting yams over a charcoal brazier...The yam fell off the stick, however, and I watched as she tried unsuccessfully to spear it, each jab driving the yam farther underneath the hot red coals. Finally, she shrugged and looked over to an old man squatting a few feet away. At her gesture, obviously knowing what was expected of him, he shambled over to the fire, reached in, pushed aside the hot coals to retrieve the yam, and then returned to his seat.

Aghast, Brand rushed over to examine the old man's hands. He had no fingers left, only stubs covered in blisters and scars, the pain of which he seemed to be blissfully unaware. This experience led Brand to focus his efforts with leprosy patients on teaching them self-monitoring and constant vigilance. Without pain to warn them of damage to their bodies, they would have to rely on using their eyes. Once he'd successfully taught patients how to do this, the "rotting" effect of leprosy disappeared. Brand's experiences with leprosy led him to dub pain "God's greatest gift to mankind."

PAIN AS PROTECTOR

In medicine, when we treat pain without deciphering the underlying cause, we are making a grievous error. It's like shutting off the power to a burning building because the sound of the fire alarm is bothering you. You have to put the fire out. If the body heals on its own from injury, medical intervention isn't necessarily needed, but when pain persists, the underlying cause must be resolved to restore balance. Once the problem is addressed, the pain has served its purpose, which is to get the person to identify the damage and deal with it.

When you get a small cut on your skin, you heal quickly and often with no visible mark. There may be a lesson to learn from this injury, such as *avoid sharp objects*. A deep wound, on the other hand, usually stays with you as a scar, a visible reminder of an injury in addition to the memory of the pain to remind you of what not to do next time. Pain teaches you to avoid a similar injury in the future by adjusting your actions and behavior.

"But why am I in so much pain for months after my injury?" Patients often ask me why their pain persists so strongly and for so long after an injury. They are frustrated at the slow healing process that limits their activity for weeks to months. I remind them that the pain remains to ensure that they are particularly careful around that part of the body so that it can heal completely.

When we see someone with a lot of scars, we infer that they have endured a lot of pain in their lives and that they are wiser and more experienced as a result. Scar tissue is used as a metaphor for physical or psychological trauma. When we learn from pain, we call it adaptive—it helps us adapt ourselves to the world.

Instead of looking at pain as a discrete, traumatic event, let's try another perspective. Let's say you've decided to start playing tennis. When you start practicing a new sport in earnest, it'll hurt. Beyond general muscle soreness, your hands will hurt where you adjust the strings and grip of your racquet. When you swing your racquet, there will be friction in places where your hand grips the racquet. Over time, your fingers will develop tears and abrasions in these areas of greater than normal friction. Eventually, protective calluses will form over these areas. Thus, injury, pain, and healing lead to further protection through the adaptive process.

Pain helps us grow in awareness of our environment. Darwin would agree that children with CIP are at a significant survival disadvantage. They can't help but repeatedly hurt themselves, causing tissue injury, and they typically die prematurely.

As much as I would like to be able to turn their pain off in order to end their suffering altogether, patients with chronic pain need their capacity for pain as much as ever. I have had numerous patients discover serious illness or injury thanks to pain, whether jaw pain from a tooth infection, abdominal pain from appendicitis, or flank pain from a kidney stone. Even though they had long wished they could turn off the alarm system, when these conditions were found and treated promptly, they were able to be thankful that they'd had it on.

THE CARTESIAN MODEL OF PAIN

Let's consider simple, anatomic reasons for pain, like a stubbed toe or a paper cut. In his *Treatise of Man*, 17th-century French philosopher René Descartes proposed the existence of a "hollow tube" transmitting the pain sensation from the location of the injury to the brain. Fundamentally speaking, today's pain specialists concur with Descartes in that they believe:

1. Nerves detect a painful sensation.

2. Those nerves transmit a pain signal to the brain.

3. By interrupting that signal we can stop the perception of pain.

Thus, we inject substances or prescribe medications that reduce a nerve's ability to transmit pain to achieve pain reduction.

This model works quite well for physical pain, or pain "with a cause." It leads us to seek out a focal, physical source of pain and treat it. However, the Cartesian model fails miserably when dealing with the psychological aspects of pain. For example, a person on a battlefield can sustain a horrific injury and perceive little or no pain and then experience agony in the hospital afterward during a simple needle injection. (We'll cover this idea more in Chapter 4.)

If we identify a physical pain generator, like an area of inflammation, we can treat it through a combination of techniques with the goal of improving the patient's functionality and reducing the level of pain with the lowest-risk intervention. When we can't find a clear pain generator, we come to the conclusion that the nervous system is sending a false alarm and we attempt to tone down the general sensitivity of the pain signaling system.

While Descartes was in many ways a visionary when it comes to pain, our ideas on the subject have evolved substantially since the 1600s. Patrick Wall, mentioned earlier, and Canadian psychologist Ronald Melzack proposed the gate control theory of pain in 1965. They described a series of nerve pathways (peripheral, spinal cord, and brain) that allow us to perceive pain. According to their theory, while a pain signal is transmitted, there is potential for gates to be opened along these pathways, allowing for modulation of the intensity of the pain signal.

Although there are shortcomings in the gate control theory of pain, there are some benefits to this conceptual model over the simple Cartesian view of simple circuits that are either on or off. More recently, others have proposed a multidimensional model of pain in which three distinct areas combine to form one perception of pain: sensory (what we physically feel as pain), affective (how we feel emotionally about that pain), and cognitive (what we ultimately think about the pain based on our value system, cultural context, and so on).

None of these models perfectly describe how we perceive pain, but each sheds some light on a phenomenally complex area of human experience.

THE EXPECTATIONS AND GOALS OF PAIN TREATMENT

Like detectives searching for clues, pain specialists study diagnostic results and perform clinical exams to solve the mystery of a patient's pain. We ask ourselves, "Is the pain adaptive or maladaptive?" Pain is anything but simple. For one thing, we know that the mind can amplify or reduce pain. For example, anxiety about pain or depression because of pain can amplify the perception of that pain. This suggests that developing mental resilience to anxiety and depression might reduce the sensation of pain and, in fact, this has proven to be the case. In fact, simply by engaging ourselves in other activities—work, sports, reading—we occupy more of our brain's bandwidth and measurably reduce the severity of the pain we experience.

We must be careful not to treat pain in isolation unless we've already looked for the underlying cause. We must remember that pain is first and foremost a symptom, an adaptive quality, and to listen to it. Our job is to search for an underlying cause in treating pain. To treat pain as an isolated entity is to risk missing a warning sign that our body is trying to send us.

It's true that once an acute injury has healed or stabilized, the pain may become chronic. In many cases, we are treating the chronic pain as a separate entity from acute pain. But I would argue that even when pain is chronic, we can achieve success with a multi-modal strategy to manage it as well as to attack the focal source of pain.

THE PROCESS OF REVERSING PAIN

In 2004, I was completing my pain fellowship at Brigham and Women's Hospital in Boston. The Red Sox hadn't won the World Series since 1918. Fans believed that Babe Ruth, nicknamed "The Great Bambino," had cursed their team when he was traded to the Yankees. As a result, the Sox would never win the World Series. That October, they defied the curse of the Bambino.

While the city was still buzzing with excitement from the win, I was walking along the Charles River and saw that someone had vandalized a sign on Storrow Drive. The sign had said "Reverse Curve" but someone had changed it to say "Reverse the Curse." This got me thinking. In some ways, we have been conditioned to view pain as a curse, as something to avoid. If we find ourselves cursed with pain, there is a systematic process to try to reverse it.

Pain is both a positive and a negative. *Pain* starts with a positive (P), specifically the absence of pain. Then, through an accident (A) or injury (I), it ends up being a negative (N). This negative state has two dimensions, the injury and the unpleasantness of the pain.

Once you have P.A.I.N.[2], you can literally turn the word around to use it as a model to grow from the painful experience and build resilience. By doing so, you turn a negative into a positive:

N. Define the *negative* experience by identifying the source of the pain.

---

2   The Red Sox World Series win in 2004 and the vandalized sign on Storrow Drive inspired me to come up with the Reverse The Pain model.

I. *Intervene* by addressing the source of the pain.

A. *Assess* the response.

P. Attain a *positive* result.

You may not know it, but you already use this model on a daily basis. For example, when you touch a hot object, you instantly withdraw your hand because of the pain. The feeling of an ankle sprain is your body's way of telling you not to run until the pain has decreased, signifying that the injury has healed. This phenomenon is a form of adjustment to the painful experience so you can protect yourself from re-injury.

Let's walk through the steps of reversing the pain of an ankle sprain:

N: The *negative* is the painful sprained ankle. To fully understand the negative starting point, you may need to visit a doctor for a complete diagnosis.

I: *Intervene* and ice the ankle to decrease swelling and inflammation. Consider rest, ice, compression, elevation, and anti-inflammatories. Again, your doctor can help you understand the best course of intervention.

A: *Assess* the response of your intervention. Are you improving? If so, continue conservative treatment. If not, see a sports medicine or orthopedic physician for additional options.

P: The *positive* result. After your intervention, your ankle is healed and you are back to your normal activities without limitations. From this positive state, you might also have learned more about your body's limitations, ways to prevent future sprains, and exercises to strengthen your ankle or adjust your stride.

There are no easy answers or quick fixes, but if you try to apply this "reverse the pain" model the next time you struggle with pain, it will help you become more systematic and effective about processing, recovering from, and growing from that painful experience.

HOW TO APPROACH YOUR PAIN

Apply a methodical approach to managing your pain. When science fails to give you a complete explanation for a phenomenon, rely on observation. After repeated observation, take what you see and construct a model. With the help of your doctor, you can take that model and test it to see if it holds true in practice. Together, you can study the results of your trials and use statistics to see if there truly is an effect and, if so, how powerful it is.

As Eckhart Tolle suggests in *A New Earth: Awakening To Your Life's Purpose,* say to yourself, "Here is the pain, and here are my thoughts around it." You start to put the pain in perspective.

I would encourage you to find the sources of pain in your own life experiences and learn from them. Reversing the pain can facilitate this process. We know that withdrawing reflexively from a painful situation may confer a survival advantage and is an automatic reaction. According to Isaac Newton, every action has an equal and opposite reaction. In a way, pain is a force of nature, causing you to reflexively back away from a bad stimulus in proportion to the size of that stimulus, keeping you safe. Taking this same reflex and using it to consciously channel painful experiences into something meaningful will, over time, produce an automatic reaction. This feat will require some adjustments in how you consciously (and perhaps subconsciously) process pain, but the resulting learned mechanism will contribute heavily to your survival as a human being.

For example, anterior cruciate ligament (ACL) tears are a common sports injury. The pain from an ACL injury alerts the athlete to a problem. Surgical repair is performed. Knee rehabilitation occurs post-operatively. The knee heals.

Pain is an important part of every step of this healing process. The knee hurts and reminds us we can't go running or resume sports right away. Much like the pain of a healing ulceration or laceration, pain reminds us not to touch the area; if we get close, it hurts, and we back off. Pain protects you from the risk of an infection or increased scarring in this case. Pain is a helpful reminder not to push ourselves too early while an injury is still healing, or we can potentially worsen it or set ourselves back.

PAIN, INFLAMMATION, AND PERIPHERAL SENSITIZATION

We now know that there is a clear link between pain and inflammation. In fact, the nervous system, including pain, and the immune system, which causes inflammation, coordinate their activities. When bacteria invade your body, they can directly cause pain when their work is detected by *nociceptors*, pain-sensing neurons. The immune system can also detect these invaders and respond by coordinating cells to fight them off. Both immune cells and sensory neurons lurk near the places bacteria commonly invade, ready to pounce when the nervous system sounds the alarm. The result? You guessed it: inflammation.

Peripheral sensitization occurs when the pain signal from the injury is amplified, driven by ongoing pain and inflammation. To explain this, think of an infected tooth, causing your entire jaw to hurt. The pain signal affects a larger area than just your tooth as a result of peripheral sensitization. The way this works might graphically look something like this:

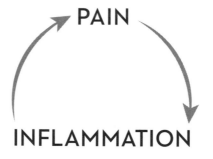

PAIN

INFLAMMATION

Two important aspects contributing to peripheral sensitization are pain and inflammation. In particular, the two effects feed into each other, which I believe forms the circular feedback loop that drives this phenomenon. If the injury heals, then things return to normal in most cases. But in some instances, persistent pain causes wind-up, leading to central sensitization, which is how the body adjusts to the perception of ongoing pain.

(For more on wind-up and central sensitization, see Chapter 1.) If your body is warning you of an ongoing injury, it will continuously sound the alarm, whether or not it is warranted. If your body senses that you will ignore the alarm, it will lower the threshold for the alarm, so with time, even the slightest pressure will elicit a painful signal. In effect, the pain alarm will become more sensitive, and you will become more sensitized to certain movements or stimuli.

To help explain wind-up and central sensitization, I will use an interesting case reported by D. W. Wheeler, et al., regarding a female patient with CIP. She became pregnant and, during childbirth, sustained multiple pelvic fractures. This meant that a C-section became necessary to prevent injury to herself or her baby. Due to injuries sustained during this fraught delivery, including injury to a nerve root in her spine, she began to experience pain for the first time in her life. Skin testing was used to determine her thresholds of sensitivity. This revealed that she was 10 times more sensitive to sensations than she had been prior to her pregnancy. Wind-up had dramatically restored the patient's ability to feel pain.

Clearly, the nervous system is adaptive and can change. We call this trait *neuroplasticity*. Consider that wind-up was able to restore pain to someone previously incapable of feeling it. This should give you some sense of how excruciating wind-up can be for a person experiencing a ten-fold (or more) amplification of normal sensitivity to pain.

Inflammation can be driven by pain receptors in the skin. Pain receptors can drive the body's inflammatory response, directly resulting in itching and discomfort. In a recent study published in *Nature,* scientists shut down the pain receptors in the skin of one group of mice. As a result, the mice had a lowered immune response.

This discovery fits with the observations I have made about my own patients. For example, after surgery patients often experience a stress response, similar to peripheral sensitization, with an increased level of inflammation. When we aggressively treat pain postoperatively, there is less inflammation and, in my belief, better postoperative recovery. My surgical colleagues at Mass General would routinely observe that the patients with epidurals for postoperative pain seemed to fare better after surgery, perhaps due to attenuation of the stress response and less inflammation.

Pain and inflammation are like a healthy marriage; when working well together, they are acting synergistically to maintain and protect us from outside invasion or threats. When there is an imbalance or lack of coordination, both can escalate until a pathological pain state occurs.

To interrupt the feedback loop, I treat patients with a dual approach: First, I administer steroids, which are anti-inflammatories. Then I use local anesthetics to numb the pain. This treatment approach breaks the feedback cycle at two points, more effectively than using either agent alone.

If we learn from adaptive pain, then it can serve a valuable purpose. But if we let pain spin out of control, it can become maladaptive. In that case, the feedback loop conditions a person to feel the pain in the absence of a physical cause. This poses the question: *Can maladaptive pain be un-learned?*

If you know that the problem generating the pain is not

life threatening, you may have to simply adjust your routine around the pain, just as you adjusted your stride mid-way in your marathon. But when your body continues to sound the alarm and doesn't respond completely to an anti-inflammatory or local anesthetic, you have to be careful not to ignore that pestering warning signal. If we fail to shut the pain alarm off with conservative therapy, it is possible that our body is desperately trying to indicate that there is a serious issue at hand (as is the case with appendicitis).

And so, once more we have discovered that the body has a way of fighting back to keep sending you the pain alarm when it senses something is wrong. When these rare, but serious events occur in our lives, I believe that we actually *want* to let our bodies continue to sound the alarm (i.e., continue to send the warning signal of pain). If we switch off the pain completely, through over-medication, we risk missing the serious problem that is occurring. Here again, I have observed that over-medicating patients rarely results in 100 percent pain relief. Again, this is the body's natural intelligence preserving our ability to feel pain in the setting of a major systemic problem.

THE BODY'S PROTECTIVE WARNING

One patient, David, saw me for pain control after spine surgery. He was managing his pain with high doses of opiates but he was still clearly uncomfortable.

"Is this how I am going to be for the rest of my life?" he asked. "I was expecting to be fixed by now."

I simply couldn't find an effective way to control his pain, so David went back to see his surgeon, who subsequently diagnosed an infection in David's spine. Another surgery removed the new infection and after that the pain completely resolved. If I'd simply turned off his pain at his request, that infection would have spread.

Another similar case comes to mind. A friend, Nancy, was training for a marathon when she developed severe hip pain. At first, she thought it was a strain. She kept running under the assumption that the pain was muscular and that the best thing to do was just push through it. Unfortunately, it didn't get better.

Nancy's X-rays came back normal so an MRI was ordered, and that revealed a stress fracture. Nancy had to pull out of training and spend four weeks on crutches. Without that diagnosis, she might have run the marathon with painkillers, causing a more severe injury, perhaps even a displaced hip fracture.

A spine surgeon colleague once referred a patient with a disc herniation to me, requesting a *nerve root block*. This is a procedure where a local anesthetic and a steroid are delivered directly to the patient's spine to temporarily decrease the perception of pain and decrease the inflammation along the nerve.

We use nerve root blocks when we suspect inflammation or compression of the spinal nerve by a herniated disc. The nerve block serves diagnostic and therapeutic purposes: If the patient sees a significant benefit, the surgeon can perform highly localized surgery to free the compressed nerve and alleviate the pain with the smallest possible intervention. In other cases there may be multiple compressed nerves, in which case the nerve root block will not provide the same complete relief.

In this case, we performed the nerve block and the patient did well, finding complete relief while the local anesthetic was working. This established the diagnosis and I planned to send her back to the spine surgeon for a procedure to permanently solve the problem. Given the severe compression, we were both certain she would require surgery.

The funny thing was, her pain never returned. This experience taught me that, on occasion, simply abolishing the pain temporarily can have a lasting effect. Perhaps the injection interrupts pain just long enough to stop the wind-up phenomenon from spiraling out of control. Perhaps the nerve pathway simply stops sending off the alarm that something is wrong. Perhaps the finely tuned inflammatory response receives a signal to turn off for a while because the communication with the sensory nerves is turned off. This is sometimes the case when there is no serious problem present, but simply nerve irritation, which once treated results in extended pain relief. The reprieve from pain can help turn off the alarm, as long as there is no serious problem lingering. It also helps us as physicians differentiate what is a mechanical compression problem of the nerve versus simple inflammation. The spine surgeon who referred me the patient was somewhat perplexed as well. He wondered whether I'd used steroids in the injection, but I hadn't.

When a patient has acute pain from a disc herniation, this can stir a powerful inflammatory soup in the spine. The central, spongy portion of the disc leaks out and causes severe pain in the surrounding nerves by generating an intense inflammatory response.

"It feels like someone rubbed salt into an open wound," one of my patients said. You get a sharp or shooting pain down the leg from inflammation and compression of the nerves as well as a burning pain from interaction with other nerves. This is what has been referred to as sciatica. We often treat this type of pain with opioid painkillers, although in some cases even these powerful medications are only marginally effective.

We know steroids are effective for inflammatory conditions, so we try to administer oral or injected steroids to reduce inflammation in order to decrease pain. This is what pain specialists mean when we refer to "breaking the cycle of pain."

We also know chronic inflammation is detrimental to our bodies. For example, rheumatoid arthritis is a type of inflammatory joint disease that progressively erodes the joints and results in joint deformity. It turns out that medications that reduce inflammation can actually decrease the level of joint erosion and damage. A study in *Annals of the Rheumatic Diseases* looking at steroids injected into the joints of patients with rheumatoid arthritis showed that steroid injections slowed down the progression of the joint erosion. Other studies have shown similar results. We can extrapolate that chronic inflammation can damage and even destroy biological tissue over time.

PAIN AS A GUIDE

I was recently in Singapore on vacation. I started to develop some achy feet from all the sightseeing. Singapore boasts many massage-therapy shops so I decided to join my wife's cousin, Vik, to get a foot massage. The cool, dark environment offered relief from the sun. I sat down on a reclining chair and met my massage therapist. He handed me hot, spicy ginger tea, which I sipped on as I watched him proceed with the massage.

He washed my feet, applied oil, and then gently kneaded them. Although I didn't look directly at him, I watched him out of the corner of my eye. I could see the man watching my face, carefully observing my facial expressions, as he silently increased the pressure on my foot. I naturally grimaced when the pressure became too painful, and I could see him instantly decrease the pressure of his fingers. Even though we didn't speak the same language, the experienced therapist could sense my pain and decide where to draw the line between effective massage and exacerbated discomfort. He didn't pass that invisible line for the rest of the massage session. Needless to say, it was one of the best foot massages I've ever had.

This reminded me of Paul Brand's experience in India. Newborn babies born with a clubfoot deformity could have some of their range of motion restored if pressure was applied to their feet after birth to break up adhesions. Unfortunately, babies aren't very good at understanding or communicating when the pain of the procedure is crossing the line from therapeutic to damaging. Brand came up with an elegant solution. He would allow them to nurse while he slowly increased the pressure on their feet. The minute they gave up drinking due to discomfort, he knew he had made enough progress and called it a day. He would repeat this process every day until the range of motion was restored to the feet, using pain as a guide.

Deep tissue massage is a type of massage where the massage therapist is trying to get into inflamed or tight areas and open these up with manual pressure. There are various types of massages but this is one that I have patients ask me about most often. Curious, I went to a deep-tissue specialist and told them about my issues and problem areas.

During the massage, the massage therapist would ask me if the amount of pressure was okay. When the pressure got too intense, I let him know. Like a barometer, this constant verbal back and forth kept the treatment at the right pressure throughout the massage. Pain both defined the problem areas as well as the appropriate pressure to address them.

Pain focuses our attention and our being. In his book *The Problem of Pain*, C. S. Lewis writes: "We can ignore even pleasure. But pain insists on being attended to. God whispers to us in our pleasures, speaks in our conscience, but shouts in our pains: it is His megaphone to rouse a deaf world." Pain does indeed focus us. It is a source of inspiration for many authors and artists.

In summary, pain is needed to survive and adapt to our surroundings, and for our bodies to experience the alarm signal in a way that we can't possibly ignore. The question is, if we need pain to survive, how do we cope with it and mold it to our needs without letting it get out of hand?

CHAPTER 3

PSYCHOLOGICAL PAIN

Criticism may not be agreeable, but it is necessary.
It fulfills the same function as pain in the human body.
It calls attention to an unhealthy state of things.

—WINSTON CHURCHILL

THE INTERNATIONAL ASSOCIATION FOR THE STUDY OF PAIN (IASP) defines pain as "an unpleasant sensory and emotional experience associated with actual or potential tissue damage, or described in terms of such damage."

We talked a little about physical pain in Chapter 1 and a little bit about what life would look like without pain in Chapter 2. In this chapter, we will look at pain from a psychological perspective. Both psychological pain and physical pain are important to understanding the total perceptual experience of pain.

Pain is used as a term to denote both physical and psychological discomfort. As we delve into psychological pain, it's important to note that the word "pain" is often used as a metaphor to denote the unpleasantness of a particular situation. It can be used in many contexts.

"Brushing my teeth every night is a pain."

"Taking out the trash is a pain."

In these cases, *pain* is used to describe psychological discomfort in some way.

In some contexts, *pain* refers to the physical aspect of an unpleasant sensation and *suffering* to the psychological aspect.

DEPRESSION

Annie was a 35-year-old mother of three. Originally from the Midwest, she had graduated from the University of Michigan, where she studied political science.

While she was still a university student, Annie had married her college sweetheart. The two eventually settled in North Carolina. Annie had been interested in becoming a lawyer but decided not to pursue law school because she wanted to have a family. Her husband was a consultant. He traveled more than either one of them liked, but his career afforded their family a good lifestyle, and Annie supported his career choice.

They had three children together: Molly, their oldest, liked art and music. Devon, their middle child, was in preschool. Jesse, the youngest, was still an infant.

Annie came into the clinic where I was on my family medicine rotation during medical school.

"I feel like I have no energy," she told me. "My body is sore all the time. I'm moody and just don't feel like doing anything. I've lost my appetite. I don't know if I can keep going on the way I am and it really scares me."

Annie had a clear case of depression. During any 12-month period, 6.6 percent of the world's population is expected to suffer from major depression. As a disease, depression makes the fourth-highest impact on society. What is clear, according to many who suffer from depression, is that *it hurts.*

Major depression is highly prevalent in the United States. It is defined as a pervasive and persistent low mood that is accompanied by low self-esteem and by a loss of pleasure in normally enjoyable activities. There are a number of other symptoms that people feel when depressed including helplessness and hopelessness, loss of interest in daily activities, appetite or weight changes, sleep changes, anger or irritability, loss of energy, self-loathing, and reckless behavior.

"I feel like my life has lost meaning sometimes," Annie told me. "I feel like I have to keep going, but I don't ever have time for myself or to do the things I like to do. I just feel like I'm in pain all day, all the time. I don't feel like I can escape it. I don't think I can keep on going like this. Please tell me there's something you can do to help."

"Have you thought about harming yourself?" I asked.

"The thought has crossed my mind," she admitted. "You know, the idea of just ending the pain and all the suffering. But it's not something I'd realistically consider."

That was a good sign. She only had thought about ending her pain by suicide but hadn't made any plans to act on it.

PSYCHOLOGICAL PAIN

The pain of depression has sometimes been described as "an ache in the mind." Joel Yager, a psychiatrist at the University of Colorado who writes about psychological pain, calls it a "gut-wrenching, teeth-gnashing mental type of anguish which literally feels like pain in the body."

Research shows that in depression there is a deficiency of certain neurotransmitters such as serotonin. Drugs called selective serotonin reuptake inhibitors (SSRIs) and serotonin and norepinephrine reuptake inhibitors (SNRIs) have been used to treat the condition with some success.

These drugs work by preventing these naturally occurring chemicals from being re-absorbed in the brain, which makes it easier for the brain to regulate mood. There is even evidence that these medications work directly on the same receptors affected by painkiller chemicals known as opiates. Recent research has investigated using SSRIs and SNRIs to treat chronic physical pain.

Pain and depression often appear together. Depression by itself can cause psychological pain, but in more severe cases it can actually cause physical symptoms such as muscle aches. When psychological pain causes physical symptoms, it is called *somatization*. I recently spoke to Yager about his thoughts on the adaptive qualities of psychological pain.

"Psychological pain is adaptive," he explained, "because you manifest physical or emotional symptoms and broadcast those to others as a distress signal." This may serve as an alarm that something is wrong and help prevent people from harming themselves by, for example, attempting suicide.

As a pain specialist, I see psychological pain producing physical pain and physical pain producing psychological pain. The two types of pain feed into each other. Descartes outlined a system, described in Chapter 2, that describes the flow of physical pain. But the Cartesian model does not adequately address psychological pain. Rarely, however, do I see one without the other—purely physical pain *or* purely psychological pain.

SEVERE PSYCHOLOGICAL PAIN

"I have suffered from severe, recurrent depression for forty years. The psychological pain that I felt during my depressed periods was horrible and more severe than my current physical pain associated with metastases in my bones from cancer."

These are the words of a cancer patient. They give a sense of the potential severity of psychological pain in extreme cases.

The impact of depression on pain—and the way pain can lead to depression—should not be underestimated. In many cases, once the physical pain is treated, any accompanying depression rapidly improves. And by treating the pain early, you can help avoid the byproduct of depression.

FUNCTIONAL MRIs AND PAIN

Functional magnetic resonance imaging (fMRI) is a tool to measure brain activity by monitoring changes in blood flow to specific regions of the brain. This lets us see which regions become active in response to a painful stimulus. There is substantial evidence from fMRI studies that psychological pain and physical pain activate the same brain regions. This gives credence to the idea that psychological pain can be just as intensely *felt* as physical pain.

Now that we know there may be some common pathways for psychological and physical pain in the brain, does this mean that all pain is truly *in our heads?* When we experience a physical injury, this creates the perception of pain in the brain. Even though we physically *feel* the pain in the body part that has been injured, the brain interprets the signals. This overlap could explain the converse of this process, why we seem to feel psychological distress, in our muscles, our gut, or elsewhere, outside of our brain, as in the somatization described earlier.

Even the pain of social rejection can cause the same brain structures to light up as physical pain does. *Social pain* occurs when we interact with others in a way that is upsetting or uncomfortable. For example, grief, rejection, and isolation can all be felt as social pain. And, as we've seen, it really hurts.

Musicians sing about social pain all the time. "Love Hurts" and "King of Pain" are two examples of popular songs that describe the very real sensation of pain from heartbreak. Social pain has inspired generations of artists and will continue to do so in the future. And imagine how much great music we would have missed out on without it!

The social pain response may have evolved in mammals due to the need for young to stay close to their parents, or to alert an animal straying too far from the pack. In earlier times there was strength in numbers. Social pain may have spurred one to either conform or risk being lost in the wild with little ability to survive alone. This pain then served an adaptive purpose, forcing us to seek out the protection of social groups by creating feelings of unease when an individual is separated from others.

Say you have a relationship that causes you psychological pain and suffering—a terrible boss or a toxic significant other. You can view yourself as a victim or you can choose to interpret the painful experience as a learning opportunity. That pain can help put you on alert for a certain personality type in the future, whether it's the next time you're changing jobs or going on a first date. Through pain, you learn from the experience so you can avoid the situation in the future, or at least to be better prepared if it is unavoidable. This pain, properly understood, helps us grow more resilient.

"Okay," you think to yourself, "if my boss is a taskmaster, I need to set goals and be transparent so that any expectations are clear to both sides." This may take additional effort, but it'll be a lot less painful than getting swallowed up by work as it continues to get piled on you. This resilience helps us handle life's challenges better. It is also an avenue for spiritual growth. By experiencing psychological pain and adversity—by living through it and processing it—we become stronger, better at living.

After a particularly bad lecture in medical school, my classmates and I would commonly say, "That was so painful" to describe the discomfort and boredom we'd experienced. Deep down, we knew this knowledge was necessary to become skilled physicians, but pain was the cost of that experience.

As a physician, I continue to learn from my patients. They each help me gain greater insight into pain and suffering. I learn the most from patients who are the most ill and require the most attention. I may be up all night in the intensive care unit (ICU), but that discomfort serves a purpose and helps make me a better doctor.

NARRATIVE THERAPY

In his book *Achilles in Vietnam*, psychiatrist Jonathan Shay talks about the important role of narrative as a therapeutic medium. Storytelling helps alleviate pain and suffering.

I can't even begin to tell you how many patients describe their symptoms beginning with the story of the injury.

"I was driving my car when, suddenly, I was struck from behind."

"I was playing golf, hitting a great tee shot, and suddenly my back went into spasm."

Stories don't just help us explain and understand our pain. Poetry, visual art, or stories where characters endure suffering can be therapeutic because they put our own subjective experience into perspective. They help us realize there are others who have suffered like we do.

PSYCHOLOGICAL PAIN CAN RESULT IN PHYSICAL DAMAGE

In a study of people who experienced significant physical pain (like a heart attack) and psychological pain (like severe depression), 28 out of 30 ranked the psychological pain worse than the physical pain. One typical participant said that the pain of a broken leg was "nothing close" to the pain of depression.

The significance of this is startling. We may finally be approaching a scientific understanding of how damaging psychological pain can be to the sufferer. What do we do with this information?

Back to Annie, my patient with depression. I started her on Prozac, an SSRI. I also told her to seek out social support and, if possible, to get part-time help managing her children so she could have some time for herself.

After a few weeks, Annie's symptoms improved. Eventually, her physical pain went away along with her depression.

This was the best possible outcome. Psychological pain unchecked can lead to actual physical damage. For example, in *takotsubo cardiomyopathy*, (also known as *broken heart syndrome*) we believe intense emotional stress (grief, fear, anger, or surprise) causes a surge of catecholamines that actually damage the heart. If managed appropriately, it is rapidly reversible, but it can be very serious.

I've experienced two such cases personally. The first was when I was a fourth-year medical student at the University of North Carolina at Chapel Hill. I was covering the cardiology floor when Nathan, a 55-year-old architect, was admitted with severe chest pain that had lasted for several hours. Nathan was under a lot of stress at work but had never had any heart trouble. In fact, he was in excellent shape and saw his family physician for annual checkups.

The medical resident in the ER started to *line the patient up*, inserting the appropriate intravenous, arterial, and central lines and monitors to measure vital signs and prepare for transfer to the cardiac catheterization (cath) lab.

While the resident worked, I spoke to Nathan about his extreme stress caused by work and his financial issues. He was taken to the cath lab so that the arteries to his heart could be examined. If there was a blockage in one, it could be identified and treated.

Nathan underwent the cath and it was negative, showing clean coronary arteries. The cardiologist diagnosed takotsubo cardiomyopathy, prescribing supportive care and anxiety-relieving medications. Nathan recovered and was discharged as if nothing had happened.

I experienced a second case of the condition as an attending anesthesiologist at Massachusetts General Hospital. A 70-year-old female, Marlene, was brought to the operating room for surgery to remove her uterus due to some early evidence of cancer.

"I'm really nervous about this," she told me. She relayed her fears about the cancer, and shared her emotional stress over what her post-operative recovery would be like. Just as we were about to anesthetize her for surgery, we realized that her electrocardiogram (EKG) showed T-wave changes, which indicated a problem with the heart.

I asked Marlene if she was having any discomfort in her chest.

"No, I feel fine," she said. "I'm just worried about what's to come."

"Do you ever get short of breath or experience chest pain while climbing stairs?"

After the usual litany of questions, it was apparent Marlene had no symptoms indicating heart problems. We decided to proceed and treat the cancer. We didn't have the luxury of waiting another few weeks to get a full cardiac workup.

I injected propofol to induce anesthesia and gave Marlene a muscle relaxant after she was asleep. I inserted the 7.0-millimeter internal diameter plastic breathing tube through her vocal cords and into her windpipe and secured it. I began the inhalational anesthetic, isoflurane. The surgery started.

But something was not quite right. After about forty-five minutes, Marlene's EKG continued to worsen, showing more signs of possible heart damage. These types of changes are sometimes normal under anesthesia, but since she was asleep we couldn't ask her if she was having chest pain.

Marlene was stable, but I told the surgeons to finish up as

quickly as possible. She started to get premature ventricular contractions, a potential sign of heart injury. We finished up the surgery and took her to the ICU and rapidly requested a cardiology consult.

The cardiologists arrived and, again, diagnosed takotsubo cardiomyopathy. We spoke to the patient after supportive care quickly helped to resolve the condition. We realized that this is what she was trying to communicate to us before surgery— her emotional stress had led up to what we were now seeing. She recovered nicely and was sent home, but not before we explained to her family members that she needed close monitoring and emotional support.

Psychological pain can even trump congenital insensitivity to physical pain (CIP). A 32-year-old CIP female had never felt pain—despite many physical injuries—until after the sudden death of her brother in a car accident. Three weeks after her brother's accident, she started to experience tension headaches from the psychological distress of losing a loved one.

It was fascinating to see that a person who had never felt pain in her life could suddenly do so as a physical side effect of psychological pain.

PSYCHOLOGICAL PAIN MAKES PHYSICAL PAIN WORSE

Growing up, James had excelled at science and math. After studying aerospace engineering at UC Berkeley, he found a job in Washington, D.C., with a defense contractor.

At 47, James was married with two young children. Fit and active, he enjoyed biking, tennis, and golf. Then, over a few months, he had begun to experience worsening lower back pain.

It started out as an ache while biking. One day, after hitting a drive on the golf course, he felt a sharp twinge in his back that turned into an uncontrollable back spasm. It took 10 minutes for him to get up and stretch it out. He had to go home without finishing the round.

James started to limit his physical activity and gained weight as a result. After realizing the pain wasn't going away, he came to see me. "I've had this pain for six months," he said. "I just can't do the stuff I want to do anymore. I can't run. I can't pick up my kids. I can't ride a bike with them." He thought he could push through the pain, but after a while he just felt burdened by it. "I'm starting to think this is the way I'm going to be for the rest of my life," he said.

James started to experience hopelessness. He had clearly become a little depressed as his body prevented him from engaging in activities that he had enjoyed so much. When a person experiences chronic pain lasting more than a few months, depression often results. Physical pain forces you to limit the activities that produce pain. Depression may result as patients suffer a loss of identity from not being able to do the things that were once integral parts of their lives.

Depression can amplify underlying physical pain and that's what I suspected was happening to James. "Will I ever be able to swing a golf club without pain?" James played recreational golf on the weekends and this was an important part of his life. Clearly, he was anxious about what the future would look like, and whether this pain would be permanent.

"There's not a day that I don't have the back pain," he continued. "There are some days that are worse than others.

I'm starting to think this is my new way of life." James was depressed just thinking about the possibility that golf was something he would never get to enjoy again. He was clearly anxious about what I was going to tell him about his options.

I examined James and found clear signs of tenderness over his low back muscles. I checked his range of motion. There weren't any limitations on his ability to bend over, but he couldn't bend left or right or extend his back without severe pain and muscle spasms. His strength and reflexes were normal. He walked on his heels and toes without difficulty.

"Your nerves are working well," I said. "Let's figure out what's going on with your back." I ordered a lumbar spine MRI.

Often, I see patients with a physical problem experiencing the psychological effects of their decreased ability to function. Those who are unwilling to see their doctor for treatment end up trying to manage things themselves, resulting in a downward spiral of chronic pain. The physical pain gets amplified by the depression. Then, anxiety creeps in as patients get more desperate, more anxious, and this too begins to amplify the pain.

Anxiety, like depression, can intensify the sensation of physical pain. Doctors suggest mindfulness meditation to patients as an intervention that can help dampen the perception of pain in the brain. Again, there is overlap of some of the brain structures for physical and psychological pain.

Psychiatrists employ cognitive behavioral therapy (CBT) to help patients cope with chronic pain. With CBT, you may still have the physical pain, but your thoughts around it change. You begin to learn to accept and live with it.

ANXIETY AND PAIN

James worried about his pain and the impact it was having on his life. He could have sought treatment for the emotional aspects of his suffering, but he kept hoping that the pain would improve.

Anxiety can make pain far worse than the physical sensation alone. Since all pain is eventually interpreted in our brain, it only makes sense that it can be turned up or down within the brain. Some patients find yoga and meditation helpful to calm the anxiety that may make pain worse.

If you've ever cut yourself, you may not have felt much pain until you actually looked at the wound and been surprised by the depth of the gash or the excessive bleeding. When I felt the twinge in my calf in Chapter 1, I didn't think much of it until I saw the laceration. Suddenly, my pain level went up a notch. Pain is an experience. Multiple inputs modulate that experience in addition to the injury.

As a doctor, I have to be particularly careful in situations where anxiety can lead to desperation. This can lead to the over-treatment of the pain, which has dire consequences, as we'll see in some of the examples in this chapter. Sometimes, there is no physical source of pain. The anxiety over something perceived to be abnormal can actually create a sensation of pain in some patients. This is why we must look at pain and anxiety separately, even though in many cases they are intertwined.

For example, if you are experiencing pain from an ACL tear, you may be anxious about whether you will heal from surgery in time to play in the next soccer season. Your pain may become amplified by that anxiety.

Once my investigation of a physical problem reveals that a patient has no identifiable problems in the body, I conclude that the pain is at least partially psychological. From there, I focus on decreasing the intensity of the pain *appropriately*. The only way to avoid any pain at all would be to put the patient into a coma, which, clearly, isn't a long-term solution. Patients must learn to accept that some degree of pain is unavoidable and adapt to live with it. But how?

Jianren Mao, director of the Massachusetts General Hospital Pain Center, likens pain management to a thermostat. "Ambient temperature is how you feel right now, and pain is a sensation that is triggered at a certain temperature," Mao says. "Clearly 0 degrees and 120 degrees Fahrenheit are both painful temperatures that cause tissue damage and require some intervention. We must learn to redefine the thermostat. Do we trigger the air-conditioning (i.e., treat the pain) at 78 degrees or at 82 degrees? We as pain doctors have to help define that, because a certain amount of pain sensation is normal and unavoidable, and part of adaptive pain and part of life. Is treating pain when the ambient temperature is 76 degrees really necessary? In the United States, we have to redefine where our thermostat should be set when it comes to treating pain."

In other words, separate out the psychological pain from the physical pain and treat each appropriately. Don't let anxiety drive the treatment of physical pain. The challenge is, how do we sort out the overlap between physical and psychological?

Feeling calm and supported can actually lessen the response to a painful stimulus. When a child gets an injury, parents say, "I'll kiss it and make it better." Remarkably, children almost always feel better after we have expressed love for the child through the kiss, and this simple communication of care and empathy makes the child feel better even though nothing has changed with the injury. The affective centers of the brain modulated and decreased the experience of the pain. The child smiles and runs off as if nothing ever happened, in most cases.

Does this kind of emotional support work with adults? I saw James after his MRI. It had revealed arthritis in the joints of his spine and some early degenerative disc disease. This mild age-related degeneration didn't warrant surgery right away. "We're going to start you on some anti-inflammatories and physical therapy," I explained. "If your pain doesn't get better in three weeks, you're going to come back and I'm going to do a diagnostic procedure to see where your pain is coming from in your back."

"So, what exactly does that involve?" James asked. I could tell he wasn't thrilled with the possibility of a spinal procedure.

"I'm going to look at the spine using a live X-ray, called fluoroscopy," I told him. "With that, I can help locate some nerves that might be causing your pain. Since you don't have a problem requiring surgery, I'm going to try numbing up those nerves. If you get partial to complete relief for a few hours, we're in the right spot. I can then go in with another needle and perform a procedure to ablate those nerves using heat. That could provide you with up to two years of significant pain relief."

"If I do that, are the nerves gone forever?"

"The nerves regenerate. They may produce pain again. But the procedure can be repeated every six months or so, whenever the pain returns, as long as it continues to be effective."

James ended up coming back for the diagnostic procedure. I performed the diagnostic nerve block and he had 80 percent pain relief. We scheduled him for the nerve ablation.

Thankfully, James felt 90 percent better a few weeks after the ablation procedure. His depression and anxiety lifted as well, once he could get through most of his day without pain.

"When can I get back to golf?" James asked. I could see he was eager to resume all his athletic activities, including biking and sports.

"Ease your way into it," I advised. "Just hit your higher irons on the range for a few weeks. If you're doing okay, you can move up to your woods and driver. If you're still having issues, come back and see me."

PAIN MAKES US MORE EMPATHETIC

Pain brings us together with each other through empathy. When we see someone suffering, many of us feel an instinctual need to assist. There is evidence that when we show empathy for someone in pain, structures in our brain respond similarly to the person experiencing the pain firsthand. So when you say, "I feel your pain," there is scientific evidence to support that.

This raises the following question: If we had less pain, would we have less empathy? Yes, this is an idea that is supported by the behavior of those with CIP.

This suggests that personal pain experiences allow for empathy toward others in pain. This also helps us better understand when pain is used as a metaphor for adversity or uncomfortable circumstances.

If we can and have experienced pain, we can empathize

better with people who are experiencing pain. This is why pain is an important metaphor to communicate how an event may *feel* to a person. Pain is a metaphor for discomfort or suffering in many contexts.

NATIONAL TRAUMA AND PAIN

On a societal level, collective painful experiences shared by groups of people or nations have a way of connecting us together, whether the effect is rallying for a common cause or responding to a tragedy. For example, the terrorist attacks of 9/11 were shocking and painful to the entire country and the world. With thousands of innocent people slaughtered, the emotional response included pain, shock, and grief, among others.

In order to recover, Americans constructed many symbols—enemy, hero, survivor, victim. The heroes that were immediately recognized were the first responders of New York City, who selflessly worked to save as many people as possible. In a crisis, the hero serves a healing function as a kind of transitional object, a comforting presence in the face of loss. Tragedy and pain produce heroes as a coping mechanism for psychological trauma.

Pain creates a stimulus for shared social connections. It helps us empathize with those who suffer. Pain makes the sufferer vulnerable and brings down our emotional defenses. Pain forces us to break down walls and tear down barriers as we extend an olive branch to those who are suffering. When we as humans visualize suffering or pain, we empathize and seek to help. Without pain as a metaphor or as a means to communicate, we wouldn't have the same capacity for empathy.

DISTRACTION FROM PAIN

Distraction techniques help with pain for two reasons. They distract you from the sensation, obviously, but they also make you an active participant in your experience instead of a passive one. They can restore a sense of control.

Giving up control is hard. Loss of control often leads to anger. We are used to being in control of our mind and body; many patients have a hard time losing it. (So do I.)

To this end, I play music when performing spinal injections. There is data showing that music decreases pain medication requirements during a procedure. Presumably, this means the patient has less pain as they require less pain medication. Patients can sing or hum along to help distract themselves and change the focus of their attention (although they may not like my music choice). We also have squeeze toys that help to direct focus away from a procedure.

A study in *Pain Medicine* revealed that texting during a surgical procedure, with either a stranger or a friend, resulted in significantly less painkiller use during surgery. The patients were awake and under a regional anesthetic numbing the surgical area, but the results suggest that staying engaged through texting may provide social support, decreasing the perception of pain.

In some ways, pain brings us together and may encourage us to reach out for support and empathy. Even more fascinating, texting with a stranger resulted in a less painful experience than texting with a friend. This may have been because the stranger knew less about the patient having surgery. Although specific language in the texting was not reported, strangers were more emotionally positive in their word choice and may have asked more "get-to-know-you" questions such as "What are your hobbies?" Friends used more biological terms, presumably in reference to the surgery or less "get-to-know-you" questions like "What time do I pick you up after your surgery?" Responding to more probing questions from strangers likely involved more brain circuitry to answer, providing a deeper distraction.

VIDEO GAMES REDUCE PAIN

Video games have been shown to increase pain threshold, another finding suggesting that distraction can be effective in managing pain.

One day when I was dealing with some neck pain of my own, I decided to test this hypothesis. I loaded up the most recent version of *Halo*. I played for an hour, and during that time I almost forgot about my pain. When I paused the game, I would notice my neck pain. When I continued playing, I really didn't feel it because my attention was elsewhere. Maybe Xbox and PlayStation represent an unexplored category of anesthetic?

VIRTUAL REALITY

How you see yourself influences how you interpret your pain. Virtual reality, which can trick you into perceiving yourself differently, could be an important tool to reduce or manage pain. Remember that physical injury results in nociceptive pain from tissue damage, but that the experience of pain is actually interpreted in the brain.

For example, if you see yourself as a hero undergoing a trial or test, you may minimize your pain because you see it more as a test or as a transformative process that you must undergo. If you see yourself as a victim and feel that no one is helping you, you may feel your pain is amplified. Both of these represent psychological modifications of physical pain.

Mirror therapy is a type of treatment that allows patients to visualize one side of their body but perceive it as if it were the other side. For example, if a person feels pain in her right arm, physicians can use mirrors so, in the reflection, her left arm looks like her right arm. This has been shown to be effective for treatment for phantom pain, which is the sensation of pain in a limb that is no longer there (e.g., due to amputation). Remember, pain is eventually interpreted in the brain, and even though the physical limb is not present, the brain can still *feel* it. Mirror therapy helps with brain reorganization and lessens pain, because the brain is tricked into thinking it sees the limb in the mirror. Interestingly, the same results have been found with virtual reality (VR) for pain. There may be a component of distraction that occurs with VR. But as with mirror therapy, when seen under fMRI, there appears to be a cortical shift in the brain as it tries to reorganize circuits. Perhaps it is this adjustment of perception that allows one to reduce the feeling of phantom pain.

Looking in the mirror helps us see ourselves. But what does one see in the reflection? How one sees oneself is a key factor in the overall perception of pain. We have a sense of self that we rely on to make decisions and interpret life experiences. This self is a complex construct, and how we see ourselves is an important element in the ultimate interpretation of pain.

In many ways, pain teaches us important things. Not only what to avoid, but how to better ourselves. Pain produces great learning opportunities and teaching points. We must look to pain to better understand and improve ourselves when the opportunity presents itself. Like a ray of sunshine through the clouds, pain shines on us, calling attention and directing our focus on that which must be addressed and cannot be ignored. Pain, in many ways, is an important turning point in life for people.

PSYCHOLOGICAL PAIN AND MONEY

It's no wonder that we called the greatest financial crisis in the history of the United States the *Great Depression*. The psychological metaphor gives an idea of how devastating this was for the families who struggled to make ends meet. The pain that was part of their experience was so significant that it changed an entire generation forever.

Many important lessons came out of the pain of this economic shock. Without the empathy and understanding acquired then, the economic damage from the 2008 financial crisis might have been far worse. Pain served its purpose.

Curious about whether economists think of pain in terms of how it relates to financial damage and recovery, I logged into my *Barron's* account and searched for *pain*. I got a bunch of articles that had pain in the title: "A Hidden Source of Market Pain," "Corporate Short-Termism Leads to Long-Term Pain," "Is Shorting China H-Shares the Next Pain Trade?" and so on.

A similar search at *The Wall Street Journal* yielded "Yankee's First Base Situation is a Serious Pain in the Neck," "Retailers Gain Less from Sears's Pain," "Brexit Pain Begins for Banks," and "Slowly, Painfully, Firms Recognize Losses From Energy Deals."

In the business world, pain is used as a metaphor for financial loss. The metaphor helps the reader understand the distress that the individual, institution, or nation is in.

Pain makes people better investors. During my research, I pulled up an article in *Barron's*, "The World's Best Investors," which was an excerpt from William Green's *The Great Minds of Investing*. Green studied the temperament of extraordinary investors. In the article, he quotes a hedge fund manager, Mohnish Pabrai, who said great investors must possess one invaluable characteristic: "the ability to take pain." The pain of market swings, presumably? The ability to take a loss, pick themselves up, and move on?

The same article profiles legendary investor Bill Miller. During one period when his funds plunged in value, the stress and poor diet resulted in a 40-pound weight gain. "There's only so much pain I can take," Miller said of the experience, "and I drew the line there." Miller demonstrated resilience in the face of adversity: He gathered as much cash as he could muster and invested in cheap stocks that have since surged. In the article, he talks about what sustained him during this ordeal: Miller drew strength from his passion for philosophy, specifically the works of Stoic philosophers such as Epictetus and Seneca and their "general approach to misfortune." For him, this meant controlling his own attitude toward what he was experiencing.

I found the same general idea permeating other business books. For example, in *Success Built to Last*, authors Jerry Porras, Stewart Emery, and Mark Thompson comment on using pain to serve as a transformative force for growth. Their advice: When you feel pain from a failure, learn from it and turn it into a success down the road. While this is easy to say, how does one do it in practice?

Pain is a reality check, a wake-up call, although we're not always ready for it when it sounds. It crosses the boundaries of nation, religion, culture, race, and social class. Even in other fields, pain is a metaphor that communicates meaning. Knowing there is a brain area that lights up when we empathize with suffering or hear of suffering, the pain metaphor evokes our understanding in many ways on a daily basis. Take, for example, a recent business headline: "Easing interest rates is a transitory painkiller."

STOIC PHILOSOPHERS

Miller's reference to Epictetus and Seneca got me thinking a little bit about Stoic philosophy and how it applies to pain, particularly when it comes to facing a situation you can't change. The only way through, they argue, is to change your thoughts about the situation.

Recently, I found myself at home with a broken hot water heater. I had to take a shower, so I thought, why not try the Stoic approach? Stepping into the cold shower, I imagined I was in a tropical paradise under a hot sun. The cool water was a relief in that heat.

Maintaining the visualization, the best I could, I made it through the shower more easily than I would have thought. Maybe, with some refining, I could make it work.

CHAPTER 4

PAIN IN LITERATURE AND FILM

I have lived these last few years with the conviction that unearned suffering is redemptive.

—MARTIN LUTHER KING, JR.

MAX WAS A 22-YEAR-OLD man who had signed up for the army in 1940. He wanted to serve his country in an honorable way—to help fight the Nazi threat and the growing forces of oppression and fascism in the world. He became part of the army, and survived the rigorous training to become a paratrooper. He was assigned to be part of the D-Day attack on the Germans. After landing on the beach, he began the assault and helped the advance of the Allied forces. Two hours into the battle, he was seriously injured by a mortar blast, with a penetrating chest injury with broken ribs, but was not killed. Surprisingly, he reported little to no pain, despite extensive wounds to his chest and abdomen. He was asked if he wanted something (morphine) to treat the pain but he declined.[3]

---

3   Based on the work of Henry Beecher.

Henry Beecher, famous for his early work on pain, studied wounded soldiers on the battlefield in World War II. He started out with the then-common assumption that, since wounds are painful, the more extensive the wound, the more painful it would be.

However, Beecher found something quite astonishing. Soldiers with the most severe injuries—compound fractures, extensive soft-tissue wounds, penetrating wounds, and so on— did not ask for morphine. When asked if the pain was "none, slight, moderate, or bad," *three-quarters* said "none, slight, or moderate," and only one-quarter described the pain as "bad."

Meanwhile, during, for example, a botched attempt at drawing blood, a badly injured soldier would still complain as loudly as any typical patient. The injured soldiers were not experiencing decreased pain sensitivity. Beecher wanted to know why they had such vastly different reactions to their battle wounds as they did to everyday pains like drawing blood. He concluded it had more to do with how the soldiers *perceived* their wounds.

Beecher thought back to civilians he had observed in severe motor vehicle accidents in prewar Boston. For similar injuries, why did they need two to three times the amount of morphine that the wounded soldiers needed? Beecher surmised that there was a subjective response to pain that was different based on the meaning of the experience to the individual. Beecher suspected that the emotion involved in the activity serves to block pain to some degree. The context in which soldiers or civilians viewed their injuries affected how they perceived the pain. For instance, a serious injury means a soldier will be sent home from the war. This could trigger emotions (e.g., relief or guilt) that might counteract the pain to some degree.

After the war, Beecher in fact did study civilians with severe, surgical wounds, and found that over 80 percent requested morphine for the pain, compared to only one-quarter of the wounded soldiers on the battlefield.

I suspect that Beecher's soldiers saw themselves as fighting a war to preserve freedom against fascism. They had been wounded as heroes, serving on that battlefield for a higher purpose. This changed their pain.

Paul Brand, in *The Gift of Pain*, recounts meeting a British war hero who had blithely rescued a fellow soldier while sustaining shattered legs. Later, the same soldier found his penicillin injections intolerable, screaming at the nurse for mercy. The lack of other stimulation to distract him from the pain of the needle and the lack of battlefield context meant the experience of pain from the injections was much greater than he'd felt from life-threatening injuries.

Our environment greatly contributes to our pain perception. In a wartime scenario, a soldier shot on the battlefield could be in extreme pain but could be smiling because he or she is happy to be alive. That same soldier, receiving a wound dressing change in a hospital environment might howl in pain because he is lying helpless, lacking control over his predicament in the hospital.

As civilians, if we choose to see ourselves on a heroic path, one with inevitable trials, we may ultimately become better able to face painful experiences of our own.

PAIN IS UNAVOIDABLE

Inevitably, life involves encounters with pain. The question is, how do you view your personal experiences of pain?

Some see pain as inevitable in life and try to use it as a learning opportunity. Without taking risks (and feeling the pain of your failures) it is hard to make progress in life. Risk taking involves the potential for experiencing pain, and without taking risks in life, growth is not possible.

There is growing evidence that post-traumatic growth does occur. Catarina Ramos and Isabel Leal talk about the framework for this. Their research shows how people can grow from trauma like combat, disease, and bereavement and take something positive from it, such as spiritual development or a greater sense of personal strength.

Great writers and artists seem to believe that pain is part of life. Take a look at the "hero's journey" outlined by Joseph Campbell in *The Hero with a Thousand Faces*. Campbell argues through comparative mythology that the sequence of events in the hero's journey is remarkably similar across various cultures, societies, and nations.

Pain is an inevitable part of the road of trials for heroes in myth. Campbell also points out the work of psychologist Carl Jung, who provided substantial evidence that myth is a manifestation of our collective unconscious. One could argue that myth is a reflection of how we view the human journey and the road of trials we face as humans.

Joseph Campbell said there was something "gut-wrenching" about the hero myth that leads us to connect deeply with those stories. Heroes in myth resonate with us precisely because their transformations and painful trials are so similar to the ones we face along the journey of life.

HUMANS AND PERSONAL TRANSFORMATIONS IN LIFE

Many successful individuals often look at pain as a transformative event—similar to the tragic hero in myth. Along the road of trials, all heroes face pain in some form or another. Whether physical, psychological, or both, they must endure it and move forward. Ultimately, this is part of the journey to become a hero.

The subjective reality of pain relies on many factors. Obviously, we've discussed physical pain and psychological pain. It's clear from research that, despite the application of a quantifiable, consistent stimulus in a laboratory, there are clearly different ratings given to the stimulus, which reflects how the perception of pain can be highly subjective.

One important aspect, as illustrated in the virtual reality and mirror therapy examples in Chapter 3, is that how we ultimately see ourselves seems to influence our overall experience of pain.

When certain characters in a story resonate with us, perhaps we see a little bit of ourselves in them and can relate to their struggles. These painful experiences are ultimately transformative for characters. Great storytellers see pain, above all, in a transformative context.

Without personal pain—without taking risks—personal growth is stunted. A hero's journey reflects our unconscious and conscious experience in life, and the road of trials is often paved with pain. If we were to show the relationship between pain and personal advancement mathematically, maybe we could distill it to the following equations:

$$\text{PAIN} + \text{EXPERIENCE} = \text{GROWTH}$$
$$\text{PAIN} \times \text{EXPERIENCE} = \text{WISDOM}$$

Pain is clearly an important part of the human condition. How we view ourselves is vital to how we perceive and experience pain. If we liken our own journey in life to the hero's journey in a narrative, we can use pain as a transformative tool for developing resilience.

HEROES AND PAINFUL TRANSFORMATION

Scott Allison, a psychologist who has studied heroes, says that we all follow the same path or journey in our own lives. During birth, we transform from a creature that lives in water (i.e., a fetus floating in amniotic fluid) to one that walks on land. From a physiological perspective, our oxygen delivery system transforms drastically as well. The *ductus arteriosus* in our heart closes, allowing us for the first time in our lives to process oxygen through our own lungs instead of through our mother's bloodstream.

Prior to this chapter, I've reviewed the physiology of pain anatomically and psychologically. Here, I'll look at pain and how it works as a transformative tool as part of the human condition.

I hope to define the deeper meaning of pain as reflected in our heroic myths and in the stories of real-life heroes. Do we as individuals face our own hero's journey and its transformative potential and embrace the trials we face? Or do we ignore the call to adventure? A rite of passage is a more formal representation of a life transformation, and usually involves entry to a group or society or a different phase of life with a shared bond or shared experience. There are often painful rituals involved in some cases, to mark the rite of passage. For example, you have both fraternity hazing rituals and the Xhosas' tribal initiation into manhood involving circumcision without anesthesia.

If pain is so important to our development, why do so many of us consciously seek to avoid it? It's unpleasant—a good reason—but the shocking aspect of pain may actually present us with an important opportunity to use it as a transformative tool.

What if you don't want to consciously accept pain in life? Although we have conquered many illnesses in modern medicine, I don't believe we understand enough about the science of pain to be able to live life without experiencing it. Trying to seek out true painlessness could lead to dire consequences. We have to find a happy medium, a balance between managing the pain we have without totally turning it off. I believe changing our perspective on pain can help us achieve better balance in this regard.

I can't think of a single story that doesn't involve pain. In fact, pain is often a source of inspiration for artists. Perhaps some of the adversity they have faced consciously or unconsciously led to their pursuit of artistic expression. I have always believed that art gives us messages that convey meaning or comment on some aspect of the world we live in. Great artists have conveyed meaning by creating a piece of work to give meaning and a message to the world. Vincent van Gogh and John Milton are just a couple of examples.

Art has the ability to convey how an artist or writer sees or interprets the human condition and the state of the world. In this way, I've spent time over the years appreciating certain stories told in books or film that have characters that experience pain, which is used by many artists as a form of character development.

Certain works have resonated with me for the messages they relay through characters' painful experiences. To connect these back to reality, I've tried to draw some connections to the pain experienced by real-life heroes, and the personal transformations they went through. By no means is this an in-depth character analysis. I simply hope to point out some common themes with regard to painful yet transformative experiences.

THE ODYSSEY

In Homer's *Odyssey*, the hero Odysseus spends 10 years trying to return home to his wife and family after fighting in the Trojan War. There are many references to pain along the way.

When Homer opens the story, he invokes the muse of epic poetry to help him tell the story of the man who has experienced pain and hardship along his journey home after the Trojan War:

> *Sing to me of the man, Muse, the man of twists and turns ...*
> *driven time and again off course, once he had plundered*
> *the hallowed heights of Troy.*
> *Many cities of men he saw and learned their minds,*
> *many pains he suffered, heartsick on the open sea,*
> *fighting to save his life and bring his comrades home.*

Books 1 through 4 tell the coming-of-age story of Telemachus, the son of Odysseus, as he struggles to protect the kingdom of Ithaca from suitors who, on the assumption of his father's death, want to marry Penelope, Odysseus's wife. Marrying Penelope would allow them to rule the kingdom. Telemachus asks King Nestor to locate Odysseus or confirm his death:

That's why I've come to plead before you now,
if you can tell me about his cruel death:
perhaps you saw him die with your own eyes
or heard the wanderer's end from someone else.
More than all other men, that man was born for pain.
Don't soften a thing, from pity, respect for me—
tell me, clearly, all your eyes have witnessed.

In this passage, Telemachus talks about Odysseus's tolerance for pain, and with it suggests that death, if it had occurred, would have been confronted by Odysseus without a lot of suffering. In other words, he asks for the story to be told to him straight.

When the reader is introduced to the story's main protagonist, Odysseus is weeping on the beach on the island. He is being held prisoner by Calypso, the nymph:

Now
he's left to pine on an island, racked with grief
in the nymph Calypso's house—she holds him there by force.

Athena, the goddess of war, is working to get Odysseus home. She appeals to Zeus, king of the gods. Zeus agrees and sends a message to Calypso via Hermes, his messenger:

Announce to the nymph with lovely braids our fixed decree:
Odysseus journeys home—the exile must return.
But not in the convoy of the gods or mortal men.
No, on a lashed, makeshift raft and wrung with pains,
on the twentieth day, he will make his landfall,

So here we see that Zeus will let Odysseus return home but he will not make the journey easy. In fact, he makes it clear the journey will be a painful one, a struggle.

Eventually, Odysseus lands on the island of Phaeacia and reveals himself to the locals. He makes it a point to tell them about his painful journey to this point:

What pains—the gods have given me my share.
Now let me begin by telling you my name ...
so you may know it well and I in times to come,

He then relates the story of his journey to this point, including his battles with a cyclops, a witch, and a journey to the land of the dead.

By the time Odysseus makes it back to Ithaca, Athena instructs Odysseus not to identify himself right away because his house has been overrun by suitors who want to be king.

Disguised as a beggar, Odysseus reveals himself to his son, Telemachus, and acknowledges the pain his family has borne over the years not knowing whether he was alive or dead:

"No, I am not a god,"
the long-enduring, great Odysseus returned.

"Why confuse me with one who never dies?
No, I am your father—
the Odysseus you wept for all your days,
you bore a world of pain, the cruel abuse of men."

Eventually, Odysseus and his family are reunited and he reclaims the kingdom of Ithaca.

REAL-LIFE ODYSSEY

One could draw a parallel between the mythological story of the *Odyssey* and the story told in the book *Lone Survivor*, by Navy SEAL Marcus Luttrell. SEALs are known for their accomplishments in special operations and the rigorous training they undergo. They are perhaps most famous for the 2011 raid that killed Osama bin Laden. Only 25 percent of those who begin will complete the rigorous Basic Underwater Demolition/SEAL (BUD/S) training. Each individual is pushed to his mental and physical limits through a variety of physical and psychological obstacles.

In *Lone Survivor*, Marcus Luttrell relates his experience as a SEAL in Afghanistan in 2005. He was on a reconnaissance mission with three other SEALs when they encountered some herdsman. They were unable to detain the men because they were not officially enemy combatants. However, the men reported their presence to the Taliban and a fierce ambush and firefight ensued.

There was a rescue attempt, but the helicopter manned by its own group of SEALs was shot down. Luttrell fought to survive, crawling seven miles with shattered vertebrae, shrapnel wounds, and a bullet wound. He confronted the pain from his physical injuries and pushed himself to survive. He was ultimately saved by Pashtun villagers, who followed their ancient tribal code to protect him as their guest. The villagers got Luttrell back into U.S. hands. Luttrell faced much pain and, as a result, experienced personal growth and transformation along the journey. He later founded the Lone Survivor Foundation to help returning soldiers recover after their missions abroad.

Many parallels exist between Luttrell and Odysseus. Both suffered a lot of pain along their long journey home. Their families did not know if they were alive or dead. They both relied on help from strangers. Luttrell recalls a discussion he'd had with a SEAL instructor. "Marcus," his instructor told him, "the body can take damn near anything. It's the mind that needs training."

BATMAN BEGINS

Superhero movies are a form of modern-day mythology. One of the most successful examples of this kind of myth-making is Christopher Nolan's *Dark Knight* trilogy.

"Why do we fall, Bruce?" Thomas Wayne asks his son. "So we can learn to pick ourselves up."

Bruce Wayne is born into a life of wealth and privilege in Gotham City. One night, while returning from the theater, Bruce and his parents are attacked by a common street criminal; the parents are shot but Bruce is spared. Their senseless murder impacts Bruce psychologically. His struggles to understand why it occurred lead him on a journey to comprehend the inner workings of the criminal mind.

Bruce experiences a transformative painful event when he falls down a shaft and is forced to face his fear of bats as they surround him. In the wake of this accident, he becomes Batman, aiming to instill fear in criminals using the symbol he was once afraid of, and becoming a legend to be feared.

Along his journey to understand the criminal mind, he joins the League of Shadows, a group that carries out its mission to restore balance once cities like Gotham have reached a level of crime and decadence that render change necessary. He is trained in martial arts under Ra's al Ghul, the group's leader.

During his initiation into the League of Shadows, Bruce is told to behead someone, but this goes against his strong moral code. Perhaps the empathy he learned from the pain of losing his parents prevents him from taking a life. Bruce refuses, a fight ensues, and the temple where the League of Shadows resides is destroyed.

Bruce returns to Gotham City and, as Batman, he protects the innocent from harm, not killing his enemies but bringing them to justice. The death of his parents fueled his desire to rise above murder for revenge.

THE DARK KNIGHT

As Batman grows into his role as the protector of Gotham City, he faces his ultimate nemesis, the Joker. Batman clearly struggles to resist his own dark side, maintaining his moral code while protecting the city from chaos and destruction.

The Joker plays with Bruce's psychology in ways that leave Batman with almost impossible choices. For example, after Batman defeats the Joker in one fight, the villain gloats that the citizens of Gotham will lose hope once they find out that the former District Attorney, Harvey Dent, went on a killing spree for revenge.

Without another choice, Batman convinces the police commissioner to tell the public that Batman was responsible for the killing spree, allowing the citizens to maintain their faith in law enforcement.

THE DARK KNIGHT RISES

In the final part of the trilogy, Batman faces Bane, a former prisoner who suffers from chronic pain. Bane ingests aerosolized morphine through a mask for pain relief—which happens to give him supernatural strength. Bane sets out to punish Gotham City for its decadence. Batman has retired from fighting crime but he still feels a psychological and moral responsibility to protect the city and its citizens. He is forced to return, despite his self-implication in Dent's killing spree, which leads him to be hunted by law enforcement as well as by Bane.

Bane slowly breaks Batman, causing him psychological pain by plunging the city into chaos through a series of coordinated attacks. Eventually, Batman cannot watch the suffering anymore, and he and Bane have a one-on-one showdown. Bane wins the first round, further hurting Batman by telling him all about his plans to wreak pain and havoc on Gotham City, and by showing he has stolen Batman's own technology from Wayne Enterprises. He then physically beats Batman in a fight and hyperextends his back, likely resulting in painful vertebral compression fractures and a misalignment of the spinal bones, called spondylolisthesis.

As he does this, he says, "I was wondering what would break first: your spirit, or your body?" It's a perfect analogy for psychological pain and physical pain—a combination of the two helps Bane defeat Batman. The movie portrayed the psychological and physical defeat of Batman.

In the end, Batman recovers from his injuries, and succeeds in defeating Bane after cutting off Bane's aerosolized morphine supply by smashing his mask.

COMPARING BATMAN AND FDR

One could draw some comparisons between Batman and a real-life hero, U.S. President Franklin D. Roosevelt. The threat of Gotham being overrun by criminals is similar to what FDR faced with the world potentially falling to fascist forces under the Axis powers in World War II.

In 1921, Roosevelt went through a transformation of his own, becoming paralyzed from the waist down due to polio or possibly Guillain-Barré syndrome. His attempts at rehabilitation transformed him from a shallow politician to a person who understood personal pain and cared deeply about people in trouble. This transformation is similar to Batman's, who began to develop more empathy for others around him after the death of his parents.

Roosevelt developed impressive upper-body strength to compensate for his paralysis. (One could draw an analogy to Batman training in martial arts, with the League of Shadows.) FDR's bold actions, emerging from energy, empathy, and optimism, made him a hero to millions of people. Batman provided protection for Gotham City and was also a hero to many.

"He lifted himself from his wheelchair to lift this nation from its knees," New York Governor Mario Cuomo has said of FDR. Roosevelt addressed the nation in his first inaugural address by reassuring the country that "the only thing we have to fear is…fear itself." This idea of facing fears and transforming them parallels how Bruce Wayne overcame his bat phobia and eventually embraced the creatures. Both Roosevelt and Batman transformed pain—and its cousin, fear—by adopting a different perspective.

GAME OF THRONES

One of the protagonists of the *Game of Thrones* series on HBO, based on *A Song of Ice and Fire* novels by George R. R. Martin, is Daenerys Targaryen. She experiences one of the more poignant character transformations and she suffers a lot of pain along the way.

When we first meet her, Daenerys is in hiding with her brother, Viserys. They are members of a royal family that was overthrown from power. The new king, Robert Baratheon, seeks their death as he seeks to eliminate threats to his rule over the Seven Kingdoms. Viserys arranges for Daenerys to marry Khal Drogo, a tribal warlord. Viserys's plan is to reclaim his family's kingdom with the help of Drogo's tribe, called the Dothraki. As a woman, an outsider, and Drogo's wife, Daenerys endures abuse, but she adapts to the pain and struggle and transforms, taking on the role of Khaleesi, queen of the Dothraki, ruling alongside Khal Drogo.

That doesn't put an end to her suffering. Drogo kills Daenerys's brother after a disagreement. Later, Drogo is wounded in an argument and soon after, dies. Then Daenerys, just before Drogo's funeral, gives birth to their child, who is stillborn. Unable to endure any more pain, Daenerys, throws herself onto Drogo's funeral pyre, while holding three dragon eggs, given to her as wedding gifts.

Daenerys miraculously survives and the dragon eggs hatch. She is reborn, transformed once again into the Mother of Dragons. Remembering her own suffering, she seeks to put an end to the suffering of others. She is a great liberator of slaves and seems destined to conquer the world. Most of all, people look up to her because she is fair, compassionate, and virtuous. Through her pain, she gained power and strength.

DAENERYS AND OPRAH WINFREY

There are striking similarities between Oprah Winfrey's life and the story of Daenerys Targaryen. Winfrey was born in Mississippi to a teenage single mother. In her memoir, she recounts being sexually molested by several people. In an effort to escape the pain and find a better life, Winfrey left home at age 13. A year later, she became pregnant, but her child died shortly after birth.

That painful experience seems to have been a turning point in her life. Winfrey went on to become an exceptional student, receiving a full scholarship to college. Like Daenerys, who suffered sorrow and rebirth, Winfrey experienced physical, psychological, and emotional pain, and was transformed through academic success. This positive experience compounded, providing her with a desire to succeed.

Winfrey's painful past is probably partly responsible for the open, frank manner she and her guests used on her talk show. By discussing their psychological distress and pain, she liberated people who were able to relate to the stories told on her show. Like Daenerys's liberation of various subjugated kingdoms, Winfrey's story has a positive effect on people around the world.

Winfrey's transformation into the Queen of Media has quite a bit in common with Daenerys's transformation into the Mother of Dragons (and maybe the future Queen of the Seven Kingdoms).

JON SNOW

Jon Snow is another key protagonist of *Game of Thrones*. As a bastard, he is treated poorly and endures the psychological pain of mistreatment as he grows up in the Stark household. He becomes a member of the Night's Watch, a band of warriors who live at a defensive wall along the edge of civilization to defend against supernatural threats. Snow trains to become a fighter and faces the appropriate growing pains along with his training.

Working along the wall puts Snow in danger. First, he is captured by an enemy tribe from outside the defended wall, called the Wildlings. To survive, he pretends to join them. Eventually, he escapes. Snow later forms an alliance with the Wildlings to confront a greater menace, the White Walkers, a group of zombie-like creatures who threaten all humans.

Several of the Night's Watch are incapable of seeing the benefits of an alliance with the Wildlings and simply can't accept their long-time enemies as their allies. Doing so seems to threaten the very identity of members of the Night's Watch.

They view Jon Snow as a traitor and stab him to death, Julius Caesar-style.

Not only is this painful physically, Snow also suffers the psychological pain of his so-called brothers betraying him. Snow is magically resurrected by a witch. Although physically the same person he was prior to his death, he is changed psychologically. As a result, he cannot continue to lead the Night's Watch.

JON SNOW COMPARED TO NELSON MANDELA

There are similarities between Jon Snow's story and the life experiences of Nelson Mandela. Growing up in South Africa, Mandela, like many blacks under apartheid, was poorly treated. Mandela was known for his ability to reconcile and find common ground with opponents, similar to Jon Snow's forming alliances with the Wildlings to face a common threat.

Mandela grew up in South Africa as a member of the Xhosa royal family. He was educated as a lawyer, and over time became active with groups trying to end racism and apartheid in South Africa. He was sent away to prison for his actions and held as a political prisoner, in some ways just as Jon Snow was sent to serve with the Night's Watch.

For both, these were transformative events that allowed them to grow into their eventual roles. Mandela became the first prime minister freely elected in South Africa, abolishing apartheid. Jon Snow gained the support of many of the Northern Lords to retake Winterfell from Ramsay Bolton and is declared the new King in the North by the Northern Lords.

* * *

Continuing on the theme of pain as a transformative event, Viktor Frankl talks about pain in his book *Man's Search for Meaning*. A Jewish psychiatrist, Frankl stayed in his home country of Austria despite the impending Nazi threat to care for his parents. He was eventually taken to Auschwitz, the infamous concentration camp. There, he endured suffering and pain.

In his book, Frankl quotes Nietzsche: "That which does not kill me, makes me stronger." He writes about his will to live, and how he found meaning in the suffering. He comes to his conclusion during his time in the concentration camp:

> I remember a personal experience. Almost in tears from pain (I had terrible sores on my feet from wearing torn shoes), I limped a few kilometers with our long column of men from the camp to our work site. Very cold, bitter winds struck us. I kept thinking of the endless little problems of our miserable life. What would there be to eat tonight? If a piece of sausage came as extra ration, should I exchange it for a piece of bread? Should I trade my last cigarette, which was left from a bonus I received a fortnight ago, for a bowl of soup? How could I get a piece of wire to replace the fragment which served as one of my shoelaces? Would I get to our work site in time to join my usual working party or would I have to join another, which might have a brutal foreman? What could I do to get on good terms with the Capo, who could help me to obtain work in camp instead of undertaking this horribly long daily march? I became disgusted with the state of

affairs which compelled me, daily and hourly, to think of only such trivial things. I forced my thoughts to turn to another subject. Suddenly, I saw myself standing on the platform of a well-lit, warm and pleasant lecture room. In front of me sat an attentive audience on comfortable upholstered seats. I was giving a lecture on the psychology of the concentration camp! All that oppressed me at that moment became objective, seen and described from the remote viewpoint of science. By this method I succeeded somehow in rising above the situation, above the sufferings of the moment, and I observed them as if they were already of the past. Both I and my troubles became the object of an interesting psychoscientific study undertaken by myself.

Viktor Frankl described pain as something that allowed him to rise above his situation as a prisoner. This was but one instance of his transformative journey as a concentration camp prisoner.

Frankl also writes that "you cannot control what happens to you in life, but you can always control what you will feel and do about what happens to you."

I became acquainted with those martyrs whose behavior in camp, whose suffering and death, bore witness to the fact that the last inner freedom cannot be lost. It can be said that they were worthy of their sufferings; the way they bore their suffering was a genuine inner achievement. It is this spiritual freedom—which cannot be taken away—that makes life meaningful and purposeful.

What was really needed was a fundamental change in our attitude toward life. We had to learn ourselves and, furthermore, we had to teach the despairing men, that it did not really matter what we expected from life, but rather what life expected from us.

Although all people experience pain in their own, subjective way, there are stories that have the ability to resonate with viewers and readers, and in particular, these are a few that have stood out with me.

A change of perspective to view pain as an inevitable part of life may help us cope when it occurs. Once we have treated our pain and underlying conditions, we can see remarkable similarities with many heroes' journeys, in particular with regards to conscious and unconscious acceptance of pain as a transformative event.

While physicians and scientists must continue to search for scientific answers and solutions to pain, there is a key aspect that we all must be aware of: pain has a beneficial role in our lives as a transformative tool for growth. Look at fictional and real-life heroes, and you will find plenty of inspiration.

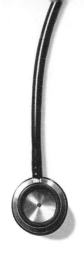

CHAPTER 5

I WANT A NEW DRUG

Bad things do happen; how I respond to them defines my character and the quality of my life. I can choose to sit in perpetual sadness, immobilized by the gravity of my loss, or I can choose to rise from the pain and treasure the most precious gift I have—life itself.

—WALTER ANDERSON, *The Confidence Course*

OPIATE THERAPY IS A controversial treatment for chronic pain. In this chapter, I try to present both sides of the argument alongside some historical information about the U.S. opiate crisis.

The central argument is that opiates are not the ideal therapy for chronic pain. In the absence of a cure for that pain, however, it is a form of therapy that we use when the benefits outweigh the risks. The decision to use these medications is very much an individual treatment decision between physician and patient.

Robin was a pleasant 72-year-old woman who had been my patient for several years. She had retired from the U.S. Postal

Service after a 30-year career, and all the work on her feet had led to arthritis in her knees. Unfortunately, she was not an ideal candidate for knee replacement due to other health problems, including chronic obstructive pulmonary disease (COPD) and adult onset diabetes.

Robin had long thought she was going to be much more active and travel more when she retired, but the reality was that she couldn't be on her feet for more than 20 minutes without having to sit and rest.

Robin's story is not unique. With an aging population in the U.S., there are a significant number of patients with osteoarthritis. Generally, when there is little cartilage left to cushion a joint, a joint replacement is performed. Until a patient's condition reaches that point, we might use medications, or injections of steroids into the knee to help with the pain.

The only effective therapy for Robin was the painkiller Vicodin, which she took three to four times a day. On Vicodin she could function, go to the grocery store and do the other things she needed to do to remain independent without having to consider the risks of major surgery.

Baby Boomers are aging, requiring more medical care and services. As more people live longer, we are finding that some chronic conditions like knee osteoarthritis, though technically fixable, aren't always worth the risks of surgery. In some cases, of course, even good candidates for surgery simply want to put off the inevitable as long as possible.

In Robin's case, the opiates allowed her to remain functional with minimal side effects. The physical and psychological benefits of staying active were simply too significant to give up on this therapy for her. She opted to continue with Vicodin indefinitely.

THE HAPPINESS EQUATION

My colleague Dr. Brian Grottkau, a surgeon at Massachusetts General Hospital, posits the following equation for patients considering a particular treatment: *Happiness equals outcomes minus expectations.* For best results, in other words, a patient should approach any treatment with low expectations. That way, any improvement at all feels like a win.

To broaden this equation's scope, I would posit that *happiness equals reality minus expectations*, and abbreviate it as follows:

$$H = R - E$$

If a person's expectations exceed reality, his or her level of happiness, H, will be negative and unhappiness will result. If a person's expectations are low, H will be positive and happiness will result. Of course, reality is subjective, so how we view our reality will also ultimately influence our happiness, along with resetting our expectations.

This is similar to how Paul Brand, author of *The Gift of Pain*, defines happiness. "Happiness," he writes, "is a state of inner contentment." I couldn't agree more. Quality of life is something that we all deserve and hope to have until our final breath. Opiates can help achieve a quality of life that allows us to maintain happiness, as they did for Robin, but we must have realistic expectations, both as patients and as physicians.

The human desire to seek the unattainable—a life without pain—has robbed many people of what inner contentment they had. As their attempts for immediate gratification leave them feeling worse later on, they try harder. This vicious cycle has led to an opiate epidemic in the United States.

There were 28,647 opiate-related deaths in the United States in 2014; approximately one-half of these involved prescription (i.e., those prescribed for medical purposes) opiate painkillers. (An example of an illicit opiate would be heroin, for example.) In 2015, the death toll from opiates in the U.S. exceeded a whopping 33,000. The rate of opioid-related overdoses has tripled from 2000 to 2014. According to the Centers for Disease Control and Prevention (CDC), prescription painkillers are a driving force for this increase.

Opiates are the most commonly prescribed class of drugs in the United States. Over 30 percent of Americans report some form of acute or chronic pain. Although many agree on the benefits of using opiates for controlling acute pain, the benefits of opiates for chronic, non-cancer pain are in debate.

The only way for a person to increase the R part of the happiness equation—reality—is to change his or her perspective. Ironically, this is what drug abusers hope to do by achieving a high. It's no coincidence that people suffering from psychological pain often also turn to opiates to deaden their negative feelings by trying to experience euphoria from the drug. Despite the prevalence of opiate use, altering one's perception of reality via drugs is not an ideal long-term solution, no matter what kind of pain a person experiences.

Let's look at the R in the happiness equation from the

opposite point of view. If overly high expectations can result in unhappiness, which can manifest itself as physical or psychological pain, then the inverse is also true. If a person lowers his or her expectations, it's possible to increase happiness without making any changes to reality.

THE OPIATE REALITY

The United States is home to approximately 5 percent of the world's population, yet we use 80 percent of the world's opiates. How did this happen? Are we leading the rest of the world in compassionate use of these medications for pain, or are we traveling down the wrong road?

The consequences of using opiates for treatment of pain are the potential for misuse. This leads to side effects as well as potentially fatal overdoses.

Pain is a guiding force in life, like gravity, something for each of us to overcome and manage in our own way. If we didn't have pain, we would not have the alarm system that notifies us when we've hurt ourselves. If we don't learn to manage it, we miss out on the positive, adaptive qualities of pain. Pain can be a valuable opportunity for learning and transformation. We must work through our pain or risk grave consequences.

Of course, the causes of the opiate epidemic are not that simple. Over the past few decades, societal changes have brewed a perfect storm that has supported opiate dependence in the United States:

- A higher standard of living, along with advances in medicine and science.

- The cultural belief that one can live their life without experiencing pain, a belief on the rise since anesthesia was discovered in the 1800s.

- A profit-driven pharmaceutical industry using aggressive marketing practices to convince physicians to use opiates for chronic pain.

- A greater emphasis on compassionate care, preferring suboptimal treatments with marginal benefits over doing nothing at all. This translates into more opiate use because there is often no cure for chronic pain.

THE DOCTOR PROBLEM

Opiates for pain management tend to become less effective over time, meaning a higher dose is needed to achieve the desired effect. This is called *tolerance*. Despite this pitfall, there are individuals with chronic pain who need opiates to function at a basic level. The decision to use opiates for pain treatment is very much an individual decision made by a practitioner after thoroughly evaluating the medical risks of the drug and a patient's condition and quality of life.

Even though we can discuss statistics and trends, it is very hard to make general statements about the treatment of pain using opiates—in fact, this very topic is hotly debated by pain-management physicians at national meetings.

Many doctors treat chronic pain simply by increasing pain-killer medications. If a patient doesn't respond to a certain dose, the solution is often to increase the dose of the medication.

Unfortunately, many health care professionals consider this an appropriate long-term treatment for pain.

In our culture, we want a pill for anything that ails us. This means we rack up prescription medicines pretty fast. However, treating something like blood pressure is objective: We have a systolic and diastolic number to guide our therapy.

With pain, treatment is far from objective. In fact, we often ask the patient to give us a number on a scale of 0 to 10. When people indicate their pain is approaching a 10, we throw opiates at them. It's easy to get caught in the subjective trap of pain, no matter how good our intentions are. This is how the situation can easily spiral out of control with opiates.

DOCTORS PROSECUTED FOR OPIATE OVERPRESCRIBING

Doctors are not protected from prosecution when harm comes from prescribing too many opiates, regardless of our intentions. In 2004, William Hurwitz, a pain management specialist in McLean, Virginia, was convicted of over 50 counts of distribution of narcotics, including drug trafficking and racketeering.

After his conviction, Hurwitz continued to insist he'd only been engaged in legitimate treatment of chronic pain in his patients. At a 2007 retrial, many of Hurwitz's convictions were overturned—the judge concluded that the legitimate practice of medicine was too difficult to establish within a court of law—but the doctor was still found guilty of 16 counts of drug trafficking.

While experts may debate whether Hurwitz's actions were appropriate, his behavior was representative of a U.S. trend toward more compassionate treatment of chronic pain through high-dose opiate medications. Prosecutors started to aggressively go after doctors for overprescribing opiates, when in certain cases patients were duping their doctors into prescribing high-dose narcotics and then diverting them to the black market.

In 2011, Massachusetts physician Joseph Zolot and his nurse practitioner Lisa Pliner were indicted for overprescribing painkillers to six patients between 2004 and 2006. Prosecutors argued that Zolot and Pliner had recklessly dispensed these narcotics without legitimate medical purpose. The two faced up to 20 years in prison for each potential offense.

The doctor and nurse stated that they were not responsible for their patients' subsequent abuses and the jury unanimously agreed—they were acquitted in 2015. A subsequent article in *The Wall Street Journal* stated that "the jury's rebuke is not likely to end the harassment of physicians who specialize in pain management."

Clearly, there is a balance that must be achieved when managing chronic pain. Opiates remain an option, but their role has become limited as the risks of opioid overdoses and overprescribing have become apparent.

EXPECTATIONS AROUND PAIN AND OPIATES

I was chatting with my colleague, Mark Coleman, about the day-to-day issues we face as pain management specialists. Coleman, a tall doctor with a baritone voice and an unhurried manner, witnessed the rise in opiate prescribing in the late 1990s.

"Now patients have an expectation that if they sprain an ankle or have tendinitis, they will be prescribed Percocet," he told me. "It wasn't that way when I was growing up—we would just take ibuprofen and ice it. Pain is portrayed so negatively by the media, people get scared of it and believe it must always be treated. That leads to overtreatment. When you hear [about] 'the war on pain,' a patient thinks, 'I have pain, so I need to attack it with every means possible.' That's just not the case."

I also spoke to Navin Singh, a plastic surgeon in the Washington, D.C., metro area, about his treatment of pain after surgery. Singh, a thoughtful and reflective physician who completed surgical training at Johns Hopkins, shared that most of his patients undergo elective procedures and are not in pain prior to the procedure.

"Expectations around pain are different with my patients since most of them are not having surgery to correct a painful condition," he explained. "They are having elective cosmetic surgery. My patients are trying to improve their appearance, not trying to correct a life-threatening surgical condition. If they were having surgery to remove a tumor, most people in my experience welcome the pain because it's the price they pay for a possible cure."

For Singh, it's all about setting appropriate expectations: "I make it very clear to the patient that they will be in pain for two days after their surgery. They will dislike me for those two days, and then they will sing my praises for 20 years." When patients have their expectations clearly set in advance, they have an easier time managing the pain that does occur.

While setting expectations is relatively easy to do for surgical patients, people suffering from other types of chronic pain do not always have the luxury of being able to prepare themselves. This makes it more difficult for them to cope with pain, which makes it more challenging for the doctors who treat them. Singh told me that if expectations aren't set prior to surgery, patients who experience pain afterward will ask what went wrong. Pain is then seen as a complication.

When patients are already on opiate medications for chronic pain and then find they need surgery for any reason, treating pain postoperatively can be particularly challenging. Neelakantan Sunder spent over 30 years as a practicing anesthesiologist at Massachusetts General Hospital. He recalls patients who were on high-dose opiates that came in for surgery.

"It was incredibly difficult to control pain after surgery unless you could think ahead and plan appropriately," he told me. "Planning ahead was something we could usually do thanks to the exceptional communication I had with the surgeons at Mass General. However, this is not always the case. It varies from hospital to hospital. Not all providers have this luxury."

When I was practicing anesthesiology, I recall how other health care providers would assume that patients could simply return to their normal pain medication regimen after surgery. This is far from the truth. For example, one of my patients was on the opioid Dilaudid for her chronic pain. Before surgery, she had taken 4 milligrams four times a day, which is not a very high dose, but also not a minuscule dose for a pain medication. Because of her opiate tolerance, after ankle surgery she was screaming in pain in the post-operative care unit. We had no real option but to continue giving her intravenous opioid medications right away and monitor her closely.

Only after we'd given her 8 times her usual daily dose—120 milligrams intravenously—were we able to bring her pain down from level 10 to level 5. There often isn't time to properly plan for and address pain management after a surgical operation for opiate-tolerant patients. This can sometimes lead to problems with severe pain after surgery. The logistics are slowly improving in hospitals, out of necessity, as more and more Americans have grown to rely on opiate medications.

MORE ACCESS, MORE ABUSE

Anesthesiologists have one of the highest rates of drug abuse among physicians. Presumably, this is because they have such easy access to the drugs. If easy access lures anesthesiologists to abuse opiates, it appears to have had the same effect nationwide, fueling the country's opioid crisis. More and more patients have open access to heavy-duty painkillers if they can convince their doctors to prescribe them. As expectations about pain have changed among both patients and physicians, convincing doctors to prescribe has become steadily easier.

To combat the issue of easy access to opiates, the Drug Enforcement Agency (DEA) has imposed quota limits on the number of painkiller drugs a pharmacy can stock. Although this may have helped stem abuse by reducing easy access to these medications, it has also resulted in some patients showing up at the pharmacy to discover that the pharmacist doesn't have the drug they truly need. What ensues is a frantic search across multiple pharmacies around town. In some cases, patients are simply out of options.

As Robert Wergin, a Nebraska-based physician, told the *New York Times*, the increasing supply leads doctors to place constraints on patients with regards to opiates. Some doctors have stopped prescribing them altogether and some aggressively limit how much they will prescribe. Some patients have even threatened their physicians. For good or ill, it is evident that the trend is shifting away from doctors prescribing large amounts of opioid medications for chronic pain.

While opiates are widely available and accessible in the United States, the exact opposite is the case elsewhere. In many countries there is virtually no access to opiate medications. People don't have the opportunity to even try them, much less abuse or overdose on them. Andrea Trescot, a recognized leader in the field of pain management, testified at the United Nations to help provide better access to opiates in several countries around the world.

"Many countries are limited by quotas on opiates, despite a legitimate medical need for them," she said. "Raising these quotas is reasonable." In terms of our own issues with these drugs, she says, "The opiate problem in the United States versus other countries is like the problem of gambling. If you don't have any money, you simply can't have a gambling problem." Although there is some truth to this, most experts agree it would be far worse to not have these medications at all. How do we work towards a healthy balance?

Sunder, the retired anesthesiologist at Mass General, recalls an uncle in India who had testicular cancer and was in significant pain at the end of his life. He had served in the military with honor for many years. In excruciating pain, Sunder's uncle was given Demerol, but his doctor ran out because of a quota on how much a doctor could prescribe within an allotted time to a single patient.

Several family members and friends who were physicians had subsequently exhausted their own quotas in a desperate attempt to provide pain relief for Sunder's uncle. Finally, Sunder's father, a general in the Indian army, went to the factory that made Demerol and asked if they would make a quota exception to make an honorable soldier comfortable in his last few days, which they did. But not everyone with cancer and intractable pain is so lucky outside of the United States.

Sri Durbhakula is an orthopedic surgeon in Maryland who routinely performs joint-replacement surgery on patients in the Middle East and India. "I see patients off opiates in two days or less," he told me. "Pain is simply accepted after major surgery. People just find a way around it, often with Tylenol and ibuprofen alone. There is little availability of opiate drugs in these places, so people learn to accept it and move on. Doctors in these countries also know that the risk of long-term opiate abuse is low because there are limits on a patient's ability to fill a prescription."

Dan Valaik, an orthopedic surgeon on the faculty at Johns Hopkins, agrees that opiates are overprescribed in the U.S. "When I perform joint-replacement surgery as part of Operation Walk in India," he told me, "patients are on no opiates after surgery. Pain is just an accepted part of the surgery. Perhaps they are trying to please us and not complain about the pain, but in any case, opiates are used far less in India after the same surgical procedures performed there as in the United States."

Sunder is of the opinion that pain threshold and tolerance are at the heart of the issue. "In these populations that have never had alcohol, drugs, opiates, or sedatives," he told me, "they have learned other ways to cope with their pain and accept it. But the flip side is also true. For the folks who are more affluent, living in the bigger cities in India, I've seen total joint-replacement surgery fail because the patients were in too much pain after surgery to properly undergo physical therapy and rehabilitation."

DEATHS FROM OPIATES

Increased availability of opiates in the United States just before the turn of the century led to an increase in opiate overdoses. Purdue Pharma developed a potent, extended-release version of the drug oxycodone called OxyContin, which was approved by the FDA in 1995. It was prescribed to treat "moderate to severe pain where use of an opioid analgesic is appropriate for more than a few days." Abusers of the drug learned how to crush and ingest this medication to result in a high.

A colleague of mine recalled a discussion he had with a Purdue sales representative in the early years after OxyContin's introduction. The sales rep said that he had recently been paid $180,000 in a quarterly bonus. My colleague asked him how he had earned such a large amount and he responded that sales reps were paid based on the number of milligrams of drugs their target doctors prescribed. This bonus structure encouraged reps to persuade doctors to aggressively overprescribe opiates for pain.

Many experts believe Purdue Pharma misled the public and physicians regarding the addictive potential of OxyContin. OxyContin abuse became so rampant that Purdue revised the formulation to make it crush resistant, or "abuse deterrent," in 2010.

What likely sparked the U.S. crackdown on high-dose opiate management for chronic pain is the number of deaths from opioid drug overdoses. As mentioned earlier, in 2014, there were 28,647 opiate overdose deaths and in excess of 33,000 deaths in 2015. Prescription opiates were involved in about half of these. The number of prescription opiate–related deaths rose sharply from 1999 through 2010 before stabilizing in 2011. This was followed by a sharp increase in heroin overdoses. This suggests that as prescription opiates were prescribed less, out of fear of prosecution, abusers sought out illicit opiates to sustain their dependence and addiction.

Thankfully, we're seeing increasing regulatory scrutiny from the DEA and various public health entities such as the Food and Drug Administration (FDA) and CDC. There is a growing understanding that opiate therapy is not the panacea we thought it might be. In 2016, the FDA and CDC issued the strongest warnings to date about prescription opiates.

How do we stop these deaths while preserving this valuable treatment for the patients who legitimately need opiates to function? How do we treat pain to relieve suffering while avoiding the deadly consequences of abuse?

I see the greatest problems when the goals of therapy are not defined well. If you continually strive toward zero pain, opiate therapy will fail, leading to overuse of these medications. Instead, I tell my patients that a 50 percent reduction in pain is a reasonable goal when treating chronic pain, and we seek this with multiple treatment options, not simply through opiates.

THE GOALS OF PAIN TREATMENT

Others agree that zero pain is not the right goal. In the *Journal of the American Medical Association*, Tom Lee, Chief Medical Officer at Press Ganey, a health care consulting firm, and professor of medicine at Harvard Medical School, writes:

> There is, quite simply, no "getting it right" when it comes to pain. It is both under-treated and over-treated. It is ubiquitous, subjective, and sometimes feigned. Its experience is influenced by culture and varies among individuals, and its diagnosis easily distorted by bias. No wonder, then, that clinicians are concerned about being evaluated on their effectiveness in relieving patients' pain, and policy makers are concerned about overuse of opioids contributing to narcotics addiction. But pain is part of life and part of medicine, as are patients' fears about what the pain means, whether it will worsen, and whether it will ever end. Clearly, giving sufficient analgesia to eliminate all pain for all patients is a wrong target—but so is treating pain insufficiently . . . Quality does not mean the elimination of death or perfect compliance with guidelines. Efficiency does not mean the elimination of all spending or even 100% elimination of all wasteful spending. And compassion for patients does not mean the elimination of all pain.

For now, opiate treatment continues to be an individual decision between doctor and patient. Expectations are an extremely important part of the discussion.

OPIATE REGULATION

In 2016, the CDC and FDA issued opiate warnings that caused a stir among health care providers, making us question our practices of using opiate medications for pain. Even among pain management specialists, there is controversy.

The following is an exchange between two pain physicians whose names I have left out. They fall on opposite sides of the opiate argument.

The first physician:

The practice has gradually been scaling down patient opiate use over the last couple of years, and as a group we no longer consider chronic opiate use in nonmalignant pain to be, for the most part, an acceptable mode of treatment. Even when used as part of a multi-modal regimen, long-term narcotic use fails in the large majority of patients for a variety of reasons, which we all know too well.

We largely restrict opiate use to elderly patients, patients with severe medical illnesses that have among their symptoms high levels of pain, patients with acute postoperative and posttraumatic pain (for a period of a week to a couple of months), patients weaning from narcotics, and very occasionally a chronic nonmalignant pain patient who has been on long-term stable doses and continues to receive high levels of efficacy.

These patients are clearly the exception. While I do feel that pain physicians need to be the arbiter of these decisions and I agree with the proper use of long-term opiates, as opposed to short-acting formulations, I do appreciate the exposure that it has had in the media. They're doing some of my leg work in letting patients know that the pendulum has, indeed, swung in the other direction and opiates will have a much more limited role in the future.

The second physician responds:

You are presenting a dilemma that has long been bantered anecdotally and academically. I think that your view of opioid management, as you have presented it, is moving in a much more conservative path than the mainstream nationally or within our practice. I am also concerned that you are differentiating malignant versus nonmalignant pain and perhaps gradually under-treating a significantly larger population of patients medically. This may also eventually limit your influx of patients and retention because your referral sources will look elsewhere to treat these patients.

You have stated that your practice is proposing opioid use for mainly elderly patients or those with severe medical illnesses. I submit that appropriately dosed opioids in concert with other medications and interventions have improved pain control and function for a plethora of other patients globally, regardless of age or medical history, and allowed them an appropriate lifestyle with productive work-related capabilities. The issue is usually maintaining compliance, but not abstaining from management.

Please understand that I am not in any way undermining anyone's clinical decision making. I, in fact, applaud this discussion. This is an academic issue, but I think somewhat impractical clinically. Pain is pain regardless of the etiology. Your choice of long-acting opioids versus escalating short-acting opioids is very well presented and well within the standard of care. I agree that the pendulum, as you put it, swings in extremes; we as clinicians, however, must maintain an appropriate clinical, reasonable, and rational approach in order to provide care while limiting iatrogenic injury and diminishing any negative social repercussions that are inherently associated with opioid pain management. Our clinical management should follow our clinical assessment decisions and not the opinions of the media, politicians, or fear of retribution from law enforcement.

There are many aspects to pain management, and carving out the opioid management component does not bode well for our patients or our specialty. A large proportion of our practice is managing patients on opioids that have been referred to us by other physicians because of our knowledge base, experience, and capabilities. We are obliged to work with and treat these patients regardless of whether we think they were originally appropriately cared for or mismanaged pain-wise. We can easily restructure and tailor their treatment plan to benefit both patient and society. We are the second opinion and we should not refrain from managing these patients with opioids if clinically indicated.

CAN OPIATES MAKE PAIN WORSE?

So what does science actually tell us about the effectiveness of opiates for chronic pain? The data is sparse. Let's talk about opiate painkillers and how they lead to increased pain sensitivity. Although it sounds counterintuitive, research suggests this is true.

Let's take for example a study by Mark Doverty and colleagues in the *Journal of Pain*. The study compared pain tolerance in individuals with no chronic or acute pain on methadone therapy for addiction with that of individuals not on opiates.

In the event that you aren't aware of methadone therapy, it is a long-acting opiate that is used for those with opiate addiction. The patients not on opiates and the methadone maintenance patients were subjected to a common, validated test called the cold-pressor test, which seeks to measure how long the subject can keep their hand in ice-cold water. In the study, there was a significant difference between the two groups. In fact, the non-opiate group was able to tolerate the stimulus for about twice as long as the methadone group. What this suggests is that chronic opiate therapy paradoxically lowers our ability to withstand pain. Other studies have confirmed these results.

Jianren Mao has extensively studied opiate *hyperalgesia*, an extreme sensitivity to pain, which can result from opiate therapy. He believes it occurs when escalating opiates fail to control the pain of a patient. "It's a real phenomenon," he told me. "I've seen it in real patients and in the lab. There is an alternative pathway that lights up in the brain that preserves pain and continues to transmit the pain signal."

I suspect that opiate hyperalgesia is the body's innate effort to preserve the life-sustaining pain alarm.

THE FUTURE

On the horizon are new non-opiate drugs and targeted pain therapies that will improve as we continue to better understand the mechanisms of pain transmission. But these treatments still require accurate diagnosis and specific treatment of the underlying condition. In other words, treating the underlying condition will, in and of itself, resolve pain as a secondary symptom of the underlying problem. But when resolution of the underlying issue is not possible, or is too risky, then opiates will continue to be a part of the treatment options as long as they are used carefully by physicians.

As pain management specialists, we have to walk a fine line. If we prescribe too much, we can be prosecuted for injury or death, but if we prescribe too little, we can be criticized for under-treatment of pain, which means patients will suffer more.

One patient, David, came to see me with severe pain from bone cancer in his spine. "Doc, is it reasonable to expect that I will be pain free by the time I leave your office today?" he asked.

"No," I told him, despite my deep desire to say yes and work aggressively to alleviate his suffering. "Your underlying cancer is causing your pain, which is a symptom of your disease. To fix the pain, you have to fix the problem. That's not going to stop me from trying, but we have to shoot for a 50 percent reduction in pain, a more achievable goal."

I scribbled a few prescriptions and handed them to him. He was disappointed with what I had told him, but resigned himself to it. I felt bad, but it would have been unethical for me to give him a false sense of hope, particularly in the event that his expectations of having no pain might have driven him to take more and more opiate pain medications. We've seen where that goes.

CHAPTER 6

REFERRED PAIN AND THE COMPLEXITY OF DIAGNOSIS

Turn your wounds into wisdom.

—OPRAH WINFREY

ON ITS SURFACE, PAIN may seem like a simple experience but it is actually quite complex. On the one hand, when you stub your toe, your toe hurts. On the other hand, when you have sciatica and you experience shooting pain in your leg, the cause is likely in your spine.

"How do you know that?" is a common question from my patients.

"Well," I respond, "let's look at some common pain patterns and see if we can do some tests and figure it out."

How do doctors find the source of a patient's pain? We use diagnostic scans and physical exams to analyze a pattern of symptoms. We follow skin maps of specific regional *dermatomes*, common patterns of pain that can indicate which spinal nerve is damaged or inflamed.

When the results all point in the same direction, the diagnosis is clear, making it possible to identify the source of pain with a high degree of confidence. Not all cases are straightforward; diagnosis can sometimes be very difficult.

PATTERN RECOGNITION

Pattern recognition is a vital part of the diagnostic process. Different causes of pain often present a collection of symptoms that appear unrelated but form a familiar pattern in the eyes of a trained clinician. One of my favorite pattern-recognition tools is a mnemonic to identify symptoms in patients with acute appendicitis. When a patient feels pain in the lower-right quadrant of the abdomen, even medical interns know to look for FRAN:

- **F**ever

- **R**ebound tenderness: To test for this, a doctor puts pressure on the lower-right abdomen. A patient with rebound tenderness will feel pain when the pressure is *removed*, not when it is applied.

- **A**norexia: Lack of appetite.

- **N**ausea: Only about half of patients with appendicitis actually vomit, but nearly all experience nausea.

Combined with that telltale abdominal pain, these symptoms form a classic pattern. This pattern works well at quickly diagnosing the condition because most appendicitis patients exhibit all these symptoms.

What if a patient has all of them except the fever? In that case, additional tests are necessary. These typically include a computerized tomography (CT) scan. The only treatment for appendicitis is to remove the inflamed and infected appendix, so we want to be sure that is the problem before we subject a patient to unnecessary surgery. Even trickier, what if the CT scan shows no sign of appendicitis? Do you operate based on a partial pattern?

HOW PATTERN RECOGNITION IS USED

My father-in-law was in this exact situation. He went to the emergency room experiencing severe, right-lower quadrant abdominal pain. I was convinced it was appendicitis. In the emergency room, he was evaluated by the staff physician and the on-call general surgeon. After a thorough review of my father-in-law's clinical status and the CT scan, the surgeon determined that he did not have appendicitis after all. Instead, they observed him and, after a while, his symptoms got better. They attributed the whole thing to some unknown gastrointestinal cause, a bug.

This experience made me wonder: Given the pull of pattern recognition, how many surgeons would have chosen to operate instead, thinking they were playing it safe?

I thought back to an experience my father encountered when he was a college student in India. He'd developed severe right-lower quadrant pain in addition to all the other classic signs. Despite this, the first surgeon who saw him confidently ruled out appendicitis. He told my father to wait and see if he got better.

Doubting this diagnosis and still in a tremendous amount of pain, my father called his brother, who is a physician. Once my father had described his symptoms, my uncle immediately transported him to another surgeon. That surgeon took one look at my father and rushed him to the operating room. By the time surgery began, my father's appendix was on the brink of rupturing.

"Another few minutes," the second surgeon said, shaking his head at the close call. At the time, a ruptured appendix in India carried a significant mortality risk.

REFERRED PAIN

Acute appendicitis is relatively common and usually creates a clear pattern of symptoms; both the pain and the problem are in the abdomen. Not all sources of pain are as straightforward. Pain symptoms often appear in an area remote from the actual source of discomfort. This is called *referred pain*, and it forces doctors to dig deeper to find the underlying cause.

To better understand this concept, let's use a circuit-breaker analogy. We have to try different switches (by performing spinal injections in specific places) to find the tripped one causing the pain. Unfortunately, we don't have the luxury of looking at the internal wiring directly. Instead, we extrapolate based on the pattern of pain, the dermatomes, and the description of how the pain feels. We connect the dots the best we can to create a picture that makes sense.

Sometimes things are exactly as they seem, but sometimes a problem presents as its exact opposite. This is part of the extreme complexity we face in medicine, which is why we use patterns to make decisions without getting snagged by details.

Take, for example, my patients with low back pain. Typically, their attitude is: *My back hurts. Fix it.*

In reality, low back pain is not a diagnosis—it is a symptom. There is usually more going on beneath the surface. As physicians, we process the complexity differently based on our level of understanding, our experience, and our treatment biases, as well as the underlying medical conditions in the patient.

One patient, Anne, came to see me with a preliminary diagnosis of vertebral compression fracture. Typically, these fractures occur due to trauma to the spine or because of osteoporosis, a condition which leads to demineralization of the bones as we age. They can be very painful, and when we see a recent fracture on the MRI, we usually correlate it with the pain. But, correlation does not always imply causation.

Anne's primary pain was in her left buttock. Typically, the pain of a compression fracture will be felt directly at the site of the fracture or as referred pain due to the changing stress on the spine. But this wasn't the case. We looked over the MRI and noticed spinal stenosis and generalized arthritis present in addition to the fracture.

On closer examination, it seemed to me that Anne's symptoms fit more closely with a diagnosis of spinal stenosis. For example, she felt pain with standing and walking, and relief from that pain when sitting. There was referred pain to the buttock. So I tried injections for the stenosis, which proved to be helpful, and validated my diagnosis of spinal stenosis as the root cause of the pain.

SPINAL STENOSIS CASE

Recently, another patient, Jenny, came to see me. She was experiencing increasing symptoms of pain in the back and legs, worse while standing and relieved while sitting. She found herself leaning forward when walking.

"I think my spine is collapsing," she told me.

One of the methods to diagnose spinal stenosis is called the "shopping cart sign." If you find yourself leaning forward while walking, or using a shopping cart to balance yourself while leaning forward, this may indicate spinal stenosis.

In this condition, the spinal canal, which provides a conduit for the spinal nerves, progressively narrows, compressing both the nerves and the blood supply to those nerves. When you stand, the spinal canal narrows further, which is why stenosis is more painful while standing. After walking for a distance, the narrowing results in a feeling of pain or heaviness in the legs. This is generally relieved by sitting a while, after which walking can be resumed.

Jenny had classic spinal stenosis symptoms. While treatment is conservative at first—medications, physical therapy, and epidural steroid injections—surgery may eventually be necessary.

In some cases, the pain generator is not always so clear. Since there is no simple test to tell us where pain is being generated, we have to sometimes use a process of trial and error to find out what the source of the pain is. For example, with low back, buttock, and leg pain, we usually look first to see if there is nerve root compression on an MRI. If there are signs of irritation or compression at that specific nerve, we've likely made the correct diagnosis.

THE NEUROANATOMY OF PAIN

The spinal cord is like a four-lane highway with bidirectional flow. Signals going to the brain bring sensory and pain input to where it can ultimately be processed and felt, and signals going from the brain bring, for example, movement instructions to our arms and legs.

Let's go back to how pain is transmitted, and review the protective quality of pain (adaptive pain). If you've ever had the misfortune of hammering your finger by accident, it can be quite painful. You instantly drop the hammer, and shake or squeeze the finger. The spinal cord reflex (the withdrawal reflex) is what makes you drop the hammer instantly, then you experience the pain just a fraction of a second later in the brain. Next, you may shake your hand vigorously or grab the finger and squeeze tightly. What is happening is that you are stimulating other nerve fibers that are not painful to block out the painful fibers.

The fibers that transmit pain are *A delta* and *C fibers*, whereas pressure and other non-pain sensations are transmitted through the *A alpha* or *A beta* fibers. This means that applying pressure to an injury lessens the perception of pain, because only so much sensory information can be perceived and processed in our brain at a given time. Our nervous system has limits, and when you squeeze your finger, that pressure uses some of the nerve signals that don't carry a sensation of pain. As a result, less of the pain signal gets through, since the bandwidth is limited—you can only feel so much at one time. Of course, your brain also begins to recognize the painful stimulus and begins inhibiting the sensation of pain. It also begins to secrete endorphins and endogenous pain suppressors through the descending inhibitory systems to try to control the pain.

When other things keep us occupied, we tend not to focus on pain. After all, only so much traffic can flow to our brain and be perceived at any given time.

ANOTHER SPINAL NERVE PAIN CASE

Scott, another patient, came to see me for severe spinal pain. He was an entrepreneur, active and athletic. He entered my office with the help of a walker, dragging his left leg. He was clearly in agony. He looked exhausted, physically and mentally. I was the 18th doctor he had seen for his condition.

I reviewed all of Scott's records. He was deeply discouraged by his lack of progress and the impact of pain on his life.

"Please help me," he said. We went through his case. He seemed convinced that he had a condition called pudendal neuralgia. The pudendal nerve controls sensation to the genitals and groin area. If damaged, it can result in severe pain. It seemed to fit some of his symptoms but, as I mentioned, making the definitive diagnosis can be difficult.

In this case, I wasn't sure that I agreed with Scott's self-diagnosis. Regardless, since he wanted to try pudendal nerve blocks, I decided it was worth a try and we proceeded. The nerve block would hopefully help us make a diagnosis. Afterward, Scott felt relief for only three hours before the pain returned.

I wasn't sure what to do with this information, but I thought it would be prudent to try selective nerve root injections in his spine. These did provide temporary relief, but Scott was in excruciating pain soon after the anesthetic wore off.

Scott's pain symptoms worsened over the next few days and he ended up in the hospital. I consulted with a spine surgeon. Scott was in such agony he was ready for anything at this point. We decided to do a lumbar decompression surgery to relieve the pressure on the spinal nerves. His imaging studies provided evidence that this was most likely the pain generator, given the severity of the pain and the symptoms.

Thankfully, the surgical procedure alleviated his pain. Scott was discharged a few days after surgery and did well. I saw Scott a few weeks later. He was still recovering from post-surgical pain, but had no further episodes of severe groin pain.

"For a while there," he said, "I thought I would never be cured, that this was how my life was going to be. Pain makes you lose your perspective on everything in life, and it impacts you physically and mentally. You're not the same person. I was moody, irritable, and angry. It affected all the people around me."

I asked Scott if anything positive had come from his experience. He related a greater sense of empathy for wounded soldiers and others with spinal cord injury or other neuropathic pain.

"The nerve pain was so much worse than anything I had ever imagined or experienced," he said. "I didn't even have a concept of what nerve pain was or how it felt. Now that I know, I can relate to those with nerve pain. For example, when I hear of a soldier getting injured with a spinal cord injury, it brings tears to my eyes because I know how much pain that person must be experiencing. I frequently have kidney stones, and before I had this spinal pain, I used to call my kidney stone pain a 7 out of 10. Now, after having experienced spinal nerve pain, I would call my kidney stone pain a 2 out of 10."

PHYSICIAN BIAS

Another factor that can throw us off the scent is bias formed by our own experiences. Everyone is biased to one degree or another, and doctors are especially vulnerable to it since so much of what we do is pattern recognition based on our experiences with the almost infinite variables in the various patterns of pain. As such, the picture may look very different depending on the observer.

One typical patient complaint: "Why is it that you go see three different doctors for the same problem, and you get three different opinions?"

As a patient, this must be endlessly frustrating. My hope is that by better explaining how we arrive at a diagnosis, I may alleviate some of that frustration. To help you understand the problem of extreme complexity a bit better in the context of pain medicine, I will share a case I encountered shortly after my fellowship training was complete.

John was referred to me with low back pain and a weak, floppy right foot, what we refer to as a *foot drop*. Although John's pain didn't radiate down the leg as is the case with classic sciatica symptoms, he had pain around the right calf and foot.

I knew that a particular disc herniation could compress or irritate the nerve root in the spine, causing pain in the low back that radiates to the buttock, the thigh, the outside of the calf, on down to the top of the foot. I looked at John's lumbar MRI and found the expected herniation.

John had fairly good range of motion in his spine. No radiating pain into the right buttock or thigh. But he did have pain in the outside of the knee, which radiated to his right foot, particularly over the top of his foot. The pain from his knee down certainly followed the expected pattern.

"The foot drop certainly fits with the diagnosis of disc herniation at L4-5," I said. With this possible diagnosis in mind, we tried selective nerve root epidural steroid injections. This provided only limited benefit, so I referred John to an esteemed spine surgeon colleague with years of experience.

On examining the patient, my colleague wasn't convinced. Something about the presentation just didn't sit right with him. So he performed an electromyography/nerve conduction study (EMG/NCS). Unlike the MRI, this test can tell us what is *physiologically* happening to the nerves in our body, and if one or several are injured or irritated.

The EMG showed that the nerve that was damaged was not a lumbar spinal nerve, but rather the nerve on the outside of the calf, just below the knee, near the head of the fibula bone. When you cross your legs, this is the nerve that is compressed.

"Ninety-five percent of spine surgeons would have operated at the L4-5 disc," my colleague explained, "but that's not what was causing the problem. It would have been the wrong operation to perform based on a false diagnosis. The back pain was just a red herring."

This was a valuable lesson for me about the medical complexity that we encounter in pain management.

SYMPTOM VERSUS SOURCE

Too often physicians get caught up in treating the symptoms of pain without understanding or treating the underlying cause. What you see is not always what you get when it comes to pain.

Writing in the *New England Journal of Medicine*, Philip Pizzo, a physician and former dean at Stanford Medical School, detailed his own struggles with finding a diagnosis for his pain symptoms. A very active person who ran marathons for exercise, he one day discovered weakness and excruciating pain in his leg muscles. Multiple diagnostic procedures and treatments offered no clear diagnosis. If it hadn't been for the efforts of two excellent doctors who kept searching for an answer, Pizzo feels sure that he would not have ultimately found the cause: a compressed branch of the sciatic nerve that traveled through the piriformis muscle. After a lengthy surgery to release the nerve, he was finally relieved of his debilitating pain.

I had the opportunity to speak with Dr. Pizzo about his experience. A soft-spoken pediatric oncologist, Pizzo is no stranger to the complexities of managing pain, having treated children with painful cancers.

As chair of the Institute of Medicine Committee that produced the landmark report *Relieving Pain in America*, Pizzo and his colleagues helped define the scope of the problem at a national level along with a blueprint to address this problem that affects 116 million people.

Although intimately involved with the treatment of chronic pain as a practitioner, and as a national policy expert, it wasn't until his personal experience seeing multiple experts for help with his own chronic pain that he felt he had received a "higher-level education on the topic." His experience with pain served to deepen his knowledge on the topic in a very personal way. His personal experience with pain was transformative.

PHANTOM LIMB PAIN

Sometimes patients experience pain in a place that literally doesn't exist.

Jim had an amputation above the knee due to an accident. He had been fairly functional afterward until later sustaining a herniated disc in his lumbar spine. The strange thing was, the herniation created classic symptoms of sciatica, pain down Jim's non-existent calf into Jim's non-existent foot.

This is what we call *phantom pain*, or pain in a limb that is no longer attached. Jim had a *feeling* of pain in the leg, even though he no longer had a leg to feel. You might ask: How did he have pain in an area that no longer exists? This presents us with another dilemma in the treatment of pain. It shows us that although we can experience pain in our peripheral limbs, ultimately, the pain is felt in our brains. Our brains have a spatial map called a *homunculus*. This tells us where everything in our body is, the placement of our head, neck, feet, hands, and so on. After an amputation, the brain map still registers the limb on its spatial map, so many patients get phantom limb sensations. Some practitioners use mirror therapy to visually convince the patient's brain that the limb is fine (see Chapter 3). This helps to rewire the neurons in the spatial brain map so that the limb pain normalizes.

Phantom limb pain occurs when there is still pain in an amputated limb. It generally persists because of the way our brains are organized. The absence of the limb or the trauma of amputation makes us feel pain where our limb used to be. The latter phenomena is due to the fact that our brains still have the circuitry needed to receive information from that part of our bodies, even if the body part no longer exists.

We treated Jim with epidural steroid injections to decrease the inflammation near the disc herniation, where the nerve root was triggering a sensation of phantom pain, and his missing leg no longer bothered him. Even though we injected into his spine to decrease the inflammation where the disc and nerve met, this helped the brain decrease its sensation of pain in his non-existent leg.

MAPPING OUT THE PAIN

When we don't find a clear reason for pain, we use nerve blocks to interrupt pain transmission. By tracing the areas of relief and their intensity back to the treatments that helped, we can construct a pain map.

When we treat areas of chronic pain, we hope to relieve some or all of the symptoms. However, when pain persists, perhaps due to chronic inflammation, pain can sometimes become part of a person's identity. Perhaps this chronicity is how the chronic pain cycle begins—and why it is important to intervene early and try to break the cycle before the neural pathways become sensitized through central sensitization.

For example, I might see a patient who has self-diagnosed sacroiliitis, a kind of pain in the buttock region emanating from inflammation in the sacroiliac (SI) joint. The SI joint is where the sacrum meets the winged iliac bone that forms the sides of the pelvis. The SI joint is a fused joint but, as we age, the SI joint may shift with motion (ligamentous laxity) and become inflamed, leading to pain in the joint.

If the patient is in quite a bit of pain, I will usually try to ease the pain with the injection of local anesthetic and decrease the inflammation with a steroid. If sacroiliitis is the correct diagnosis, the patient should report immediate relief from the local anesthetic and experience long-term benefits from the steroid. When relief is minimal, however, the problem lies elsewhere.

Often, pain appearing to come from the SI joint is referred from another source, such as the lumbar spine, as in the case of a herniated disc. The strange thing is that patients will often be offended. "Are you saying I don't have sacroiliitis?" they'll exclaim. "My doctor has been treating me for this for years. Are you saying it's not the problem?" From the reaction, it can almost feel like the patient's very identity is threatened. In a way, pain can become part of a patient's identity and self-image. In one case, a patient was so offended by my idea that he *didn't* have a problem with his SI joint that he abruptly got up and left the exam room.

THE DREAM OF PAIN-FREE

It's rare, but some patients see me thinking they will leave my office pain-free. I wish this were the case, but we simply don't have the tools to make this happen in a majority of cases.

"Think of pain on a continuum," I explain. "If we're lucky, I will reduce your pain by half, which is actually a big improvement. Then we can decide where to go from there." Of course, in rare cases we immediately find the root cause and are able to treat it on the spot, achieving complete pain relief. Those are, by far, the exceptions, though.

Research provides us some insight into the treatment of painful conditions. However, it's a bit limited with regard to chronic pain. Studies often look at how one isolated piece of data influences other pieces of data. This can be very helpful when one variable directly affects many other systems. But definitive studies are hard to do in pain medicine because there is a subjective endpoint (pain or functioning), which is not easily quantified compared to, say, a cholesterol level. Perhaps we will identify quantifiable biomarkers for pain in the future, but at the present time we must rely on patients to self-report.

I spoke to a physician who had performed acupuncture on his patients with chronic pain. He told me about a case that stood out to him—a patient with chronic abdominal pain. All available treatments had failed. The physician slowly, methodically applied acupuncture for the patient's symptoms and the patient's pain slowly decreased from 10 to a 2.5 on a 10-point scale.

One day, the patient stopped coming to see him. After some investigating, the doctor learned that the patient had actually stopped treatment because his pain had become such a key part of his identity that he was terrified to live without it.

NEUROINFLAMMATION

The concept of *neuroinflammation*—inflammation around or in nerve tissue—causing pain is changing chronic pain treatment. In the past, we've looked for compression of a nerve on imaging studies, but we now know there can be underlying inflammation without direct compression visible in a scan. Multiple sclerosis, for example, is an example of a neuroinflammatory disease.

In researching pain, doctors may have multiple pieces of data with no clear idea of how to weigh each one against the others. This challenge is the essence of clinical practice in pain management. Most of the time, we deal with neuroinflammation in the spinal or in the peripheral nerves. We don't always see it on a scan, but can infer that it may exist based on the pattern of a patient's pain.

Because pain is not something we can see on a scan or MRI, some doctors prefer not to operate when the problem is hard to identify and the primary symptom is pain. In fact, I have come across spine surgeons who find pain so frustrating that they choose not to operate on patients solely for pain. They only want referrals for the removal of spine tumors, a procedure with a clear and objective outcome.

Jane had undergone an anterior cervical discectomy and fusion, a surgery for spinal stenosis where the discs are removed and the bones in the spine fused together through an incision in the front of the neck. A week after her surgery, she began to experience severe arm pain, and her doctor referred her to me.

In my office, I found that Jane's skin had turned beet red. Even a light touch of her arm evoked severe, burning pain; she couldn't bear to wear a watch. These are classic symptoms of complex regional pain syndrome (CRPS).

CRPS occurs when nerves start to overreact in response to an injury, an example of pathological pain that we need to quickly shut down before the body's wiring enters a perpetual state of hypersensitivity. By calming down the nerves before this process can occur, we prevent the pain from traveling or extending to multiple places in the nervous system in addition to the initial site of injury. When CRPS is caught early and treated, it is completely curable in most cases. But once central sensitization and neuroplasticity changes have occurred, it can become very difficult to treat.

In Jane's case, we were not sure what had caused her CRPS. The surgeon suspected a stretch may have occurred on the cervical plexus of nerves during the surgery. We thought that, perhaps, it could also be tissue trauma itself. Fortunately, we caught the issue quickly and were able to perform two nerve blocks to tone down the nervous system sensitivity rapidly. Fortunately, the pain did not come back.

In CRPS, the nerves are going, quite literally, haywire. CRPS results in worsening pain without any ongoing injury. When the diagnosis is delayed, it can take eight or more nerve blocks, or even an implanted spinal cord stimulator, to correct the pain once it has been hardwired into the nervous system.

I once treated a patient who couldn't bear the pain of CRPS anymore. As a result, she neglected her arm with CRPS and refused to touch, wash, or even acknowledge that she had the arm, which subsequently caused it to become infected and later amputated. Although she was initially happy to have this happen, she soon realized that the pain persisted and had transformed into phantom pain syndrome.

For patients with CRPS, most doctors recommend continuing physical activity, which means using nerves other than the pain-signaling nerves. This is the gate control theory in action again: If you stimulate non-painful nerves, the pain nerve gates will close to allow the others to send their message. If there is no other stimulation, the pain nerves will continue to transmit their signals.

We have a tendency to avoid using the painful body part, but if we allow this to happen, the body senses this diminished activity and starts to increase its neural wiring and circuits to the area so we can use it more. This is neuroplasticity, and it leads to more conduits for pain and eventually central sensitization. The expression "use it or lose it" couldn't be more appropriate in this situation. The lesson here is that you can't completely disconnect from your pain.

Another way to view the role of activity in CRPS is as a distraction. By doing activity, you may be distracting yourself from the pain and breaking the cycle of disuse and wind-up.

When a stimulus is too painful to autoregulate, or when it persists and leads to chronic pain, we need options to help us provide the switch to non-painful fibers. I believe we can use this principle to self-modulate our pain before maladaptive neural wind-up occurs. Most of us do this instinctively, but I believe that we can use it systematically to prevent these problems from worsening.

When a nerve is injured and there is loss of function, the nervous system enters survival mode. The message is sent to the brain that it has a severed connection. In an effort to try to recover the signal of sensation from this nerve, the nerve endings on the proximal side of the nerve start to sprout in an effort to try to reestablish connection and control.

An unfortunate side effect is that the nerve has even more nerve endings and receptors, which gives it more opportunities to transmit pain. This is the same reason why so many patients who have had a stroke with loss of function can, in fact, recover function with the proper therapy. However, as these patients regain function due to nerves awakening after the stroke, they experience pain. This is also true in cases of patients with injuries to their spinal cord. As they regain function, pain often accompanies their recovery.

SPINAL CORD STIMULATION AND NEUROINFLAMMATION

It can become incredibly frustrating to the patient when we can't find any evidence for a pain generator.

"Are you saying I don't have pain?" they ask. "That it's all in my head?"

"No," I reassure them. "I believe you have pain. We just need to look a bit harder to understand what's causing you to have these symptoms."

When it comes to chronic pain, there is growing evidence that increased activity along the various neural pathways causes neuroinflammation, making the body's neurons so sensitive that harmless sensations can cause pain. The neurological system becomes hyperactive and hypersensitive to ordinary things like brushing your teeth or putting on socks. *Allodynia* is when a non-painful stimulus causes pain. *Hyperalgesia* is when a painful stimulus causes pain out of proportion to what one would expect. Both are signs of neuroinflammation.

If we can't find the focal pain generator, we have to assume it's a nerve problem and try to reduce that neuropathic pain.

We may use *neuromodulation* to tone down the sensitivity of the nerves. Neuromodulation is frequently performed via spinal cord stimulation. An implant adjacent to the spinal cord produces electrical impulses in a variant of electroacupuncture. A spinal cord stimulator is a marvel of modern technology. It looks like a hockey puck with a wire coming out of it, and it's designed to sit safely inside the body. It's actually very similar to a pacemaker. Both use electrical signals to stimulate organs, the pacemaker for the heart and the spinal cord stimulator for the spinal cord.

In 1967, neurosurgeon Norman Shealy became the first to perform spinal cord stimulation. Neuromodulation through spinal cord stimulation therapy stimulates non-painful pathways to decrease the perception of painful signals along painful neural pathways. We typically use it for nerve-related pain, or if there is neuroinflammation when there isn't evidence of clinically significant compression of a spinal nerve on the MRI. The spinal cord stimulator acts to signal through non-painful pathways in the spinal cord. Since only so many gates can be open to send nerve signals, the painful pathways' gates are necessarily closed.

Futurist and author Ray Kurzweil envisions nanobots floating around in our bloodstream as a mechanism to identify and provide an early fix for problems, from inflammation to cancer, addressing them before they get out of control. While I don't see myself injecting tiny robots into my patients any time soon, I do believe the future looks bright for neuromodulation therapy. It may one day hold the cure for unnecessary chronic pain and inflammation.

SPINAL CORD STIMULATOR CASE

Another patient, John, was a state trooper who loved his job. He was involved in a catastrophic accident while performing his duties. His car ended up crashing into the highway barrier, leaving him severely injured. Despite the great care he received, John was left with severe, chronic pain in his low back and legs.

After several grueling operations, John was released, able to walk using a walker. He required several additional operations to open areas where his spine had narrowed and to remove some hardware that had been placed to allow his bones to heal. Although he was fortunate to be alive, he was in constant, chronic pain.

John came to see me. Initially, we managed his pain using opiate medications. Once we realized that he was not where he needed to be after exhausting all our options for conservative therapy, we decided to try a spinal cord stimulator.

First, I performed a trial, inserting a temporary wire into the spinal canal to see where an electrical stimulation might create a reduction in pain. By delivering targeted electrical signals to specific areas of the spinal cord, we were able to map where the pain signal could be interrupted. The trial achieved a 75 percent reduction in pain, so I decided to proceed to a permanent implant. With that, John was able to manage on minimal to moderate opiate medications only when experiencing muscular pain not traditionally controlled well by the stimulator.

Is a spinal cord stimulator a permanent pain cure? Not exactly. In one particular patient, we inserted a spinal cord stimulator after all conservative therapy options had failed.

Her trial worked well. While the implanted stimulator initially worked, within six months its effects had faded. Despite reprogramming the stimulator, we couldn't reduce her pain level. We re-imaged her spine and the CT scan revealed the cause: an acute compression fracture of the spine, putting pressure on an adjacent nerve. When nerves are compressed, stimulation simply does not work. The body is too smart to not sound the alarm. As always, adaptive pain is working on our behalf. We treated the compression fracture and her pain eventually resolved, though she continued to use the stimulator occasionally.

Although chronic pain might drive us to look for a way to turn pain off, these cases are proof that even if you suffer from severe, chronic pain, pain still serves an important purpose, alerting us to new problems as they arise, whether it be appendicitis or the fracture of a bone. To lose the ability to sense pain would leave the body vulnerable to injury or allow a serious condition to be undetected. It is the very acute and severe nature of pain that forces us to take action as opposed to sitting around until your condition worsens beyond repair.

THE IMPORTANCE OF MAKING A DIAGNOSIS

I have experienced pain firsthand and I can use that experience to better relate to my patients. For a doctor, this is a luxury. Not all physicians have experienced the exact same symptoms as their patients have—most oncologists, for example, aren't cancer survivors. When pain is the problem, however, empathy flows naturally and becomes a natural part of the doctor-patient interaction.

I experienced unremitting hip pain for over a year. Having enthusiastically picked up golf for the fourth time in my life—after watching Tiger Woods win the Wells Fargo Championship in 2007—I was determined to shave some points off my golf score with lessons. I took every opportunity to improve my game. Upon returning home from a golf trip, I noticed some pain in my left buttock. Thinking it was nothing more than a muscle sprain, I ignored it, but the burning sensation wouldn't go away.

I self-diagnosed it as sacroiliitis and asked a physician colleague to perform a steroid injection into the sacroiliac joint. The pain went away for a week and then came back. I self-diagnosed it as myofascial pain and asked the same colleague to perform trigger-point injections. Again, only temporary relief.

I started to get concerned because I couldn't figure out what the heck was causing my pain. I saw an orthopedic surgeon and tried physical therapy for my hip, all to no avail. I thought it could be an issue with my lumbar spine, but the MRI was negative in that area. After reflecting on my symptoms, I decided something was going on with my hip, so I saw another orthopedic surgeon, who ordered a hip MRI.

Lying in the round MRI cylinder with headphones on, I understood why some of my patients panic from claustrophobia during the process. Luckily, I didn't experience that myself and slept through most of it. The results came back a day later, revealing a tear of the hip cartilage, called the labrum, which forms a suction cup or socket around the ball of the femur bone. It's an injury that can occur from the repetitive motion of sports such as golf or baseball, where rotational torque puts stress on the hip joint. I was relieved to finally know the cause. I just had to decide what to do about it.

At the time, I was lucky to be working as an anesthesiologist at the prestigious Massachusetts General Hospital in Boston. The hospital, affiliated with Harvard Medical School, is the third oldest in the United States, the site of the first public display of anesthesia in 1846. With so many important medical discoveries in its history, some say Mass General is to medicine what the Louvre is to art.

I was friendly with several of the world-renowned orthopedic surgeons on staff, so I saw four different surgeons to discuss my options. I pored over the medical literature on hip labral tears. Three of them recommended managing it conservatively without surgery. I was disappointed, to say the least, but then I saw Joe McCarthy, a pioneer in hip arthroscopy. He was optimistic we could fix the tear surgically. I decided that was the best option for me.

I went in for surgery, and McCarthy, operating through three small incisions, was able to remove the torn part of the cartilage and smooth out the rest so it would heal. Nine months after the arthroscopic procedure, I had only minimal pain, though it would still flare up during certain sports or activities. The images taken during the surgery showed early signs of arthritis of the hip, too faint to see on X-rays or MRIs. Armed with that knowledge, I'm better able to manage my pain and to protect my hip against worsening arthritis.

In some ways, my experiences with pain and injury have made me a better physician. For a long time, I ignored the hip pain and pushed through it. When I finally reached a correct diagnosis, a year or so after the onset of the chronic pain, I was mentally fatigued and my hip was quite inflamed.

The evidence for hip labral tears causing pain is mixed; some studies show the presence of tears in completely asymptomatic patients and others show that the tears are symptomatic. I feel there is a difference between symptomatic and asymptomatic tears, but there is some thought that both lead to early arthritis, and may explain why people sometimes have one hip joint that is bone on bone and needs a joint replacement, while the other may have little to no arthritis.

Only after considering the opinions of four orthopedic surgeons did I decide to pursue surgery, which finally brought relief. Along the way, I became a better diagnostician because it is now easier for me to help others diagnose this uncommon injury. My pain forced me to become a better doctor and pain specialist, and I feel I am better at recognizing these symptoms, differentiating this condition from other pain generators, and helping patients navigate their treatment options.

This is not only a great example of bringing symptoms together to make a diagnosis, but also of how to transform your pain into something that can benefit you and others.

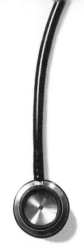

CHAPTER 7

HOW WE
MANAGE PAIN

The game of basketball has been everything to me.
My place of refuge, [a] place I've always gone where
I needed comfort and peace. It's been the site of intense
pain and the most intense feelings of joy and satisfaction.
It's a relationship that has evolved over time, given me
the greatest respect and love for the game.

—MICHAEL JORDAN

JOANNE, A 60-YEAR-OLD PART-TIME librarian with wavy brown hair, soft eyes, and a gentle smile, came in to see me for her low back pain. It had worsened over the past year, with excruciating and even disabling flare-ups. Just recently, she had begun to experience right leg pain as well.

"It's starting to slow me down," she told me. "I can't do simple things that I enjoy like taking walks or buying groceries."

Low back pain hits almost all of us at some point in our lives. The annual financial toll, between treatment and lost productivity, amounts to over $100 billion in the United States alone. Most of the time, this kind of pain goes away with rest and anti-inflammatory medication like ibuprofen.

While low back pain rarely becomes chronic, if it persists for weeks or even months, it's time to see a doctor. Most people will start off with a visit to their primary care doctor, who will typically prescribe ice or heat, pain medication, and physical therapy. However, as treatment options have improved, many patients are simply referred to a pain specialist like me.

"I really don't want to be cut open," Joanne told me. Some patients are terrified of having back surgery. This is often the first thing new patients tell me when they are in severe pain.

People often correlate the severity of pain with the aggressiveness of interventions. Thankfully, this is not always the case. It's rare in patients with low back pain to encounter a condition like cancer or a serious infection in the spine, which may require immediate surgery. Another condition requiring aggressive intervention is cauda equina syndrome (CES), where the spinal nerves are compressed and injured, causing numbness, weakness, and a loss of bladder and bowel control. Like other ailments requiring surgical intervention, CES is uncommon.

Fortunately, Joanne fell into none of these categories. She just had pain. Over the past few years, she'd found it more and more difficult to bend, lift, or even sit in a chair for extended periods, let alone go for a long drive. We take these simple daily activities for granted until we see how limiting pain can be from a functional standpoint.

I reviewed Joanne's lumbar MRI scans. (My colleague Jay Khanna at Johns Hopkins calls this imaging scan the "stethoscope" for the spine.) Joanne had told me her pain traveled from the low back to the hip and down the leg in a particular nerve and skin sensory pattern or dermatome. The MRI confirmed the diagnosis these symptoms suggested: L5-S1 narrowing, or stenosis, compressing the L5 nerve.

There are four regions in the spine: cervical (neck), thoracic (chest), lumbar (low back), and sacral (buttocks). The vertebrae each have a letter and a number to tell where you are in the spine. For example, L5 is the fifth lumbar vertebra. Since spinal nerves exit the spine between two vertebrae, we refer to these locations by the adjacent vertebrae. L5-S1 denotes the spinal segment between the fifth lumbar vertebra and the first sacral vertebra. When a spinal nerve is compressed or damaged by spinal narrowing, patients experience pain, numbness, tingling, or weakness.

I use a series of tests to find the pain generator. Once I have found it, I use various treatments to decrease pain and improve function. In some cases, the injections I perform can be both diagnostic and therapeutic; when I do something that results in significant pain relief, I can better diagnose the cause of the pain based on the injection that relieved it. Injections can only do so much, though. When real damage has occurred, it's time for a surgical evaluation.

Joanne and I discussed a treatment strategy for her pain. "I just want to be able to have a normal life," she said. "I don't want to be on all these drugs, but I have to in order to keep going."

In some patients the cause of pain is elusive. Batteries of tests, injections, medications, and physical therapy lead to no diagnosis and no benefit. We rarely risk surgery when we aren't sure of the pain's cause; in these cases the risks outweigh the possible benefits. Instead, we try more conservative interventions in the hopes that the pain generator will become apparent in the process.

"Your options fall into four buckets," I told Joanne, "medication, physical therapy, injections, and surgery." We tried pregabalin, a drug that blocks sensations going to the brain, and duloxetine, which inhibits pain by boosting serotonin and norepinephrine levels. Both work by different mechanisms. Each helped, but they didn't reduce the pain as much as we'd have liked, so we decided to proceed to a selective nerve root epidural injection.

At the start of the procedure, Joanne was positioned on the O.R. table. My assistant tuned the radio to a classic rock station to help distract and relax her. The nurses cleansed the site of the injection with an antiseptic solution while The Ramones blared "I Wanna Be Sedated." I drew up a syringe of local anesthetic hoping the irony of the song's title might serve to lessen her anxiety about the upcoming procedure.

"How do you practice these injections?" she asked.

"I throw darts at a local bar," I joked.

I could see that I had disarmed her with my attempt at humor. Somehow, my jokes are always funnier to my patients when I'm brandishing a spinal needle.

Carefully, I inserted the smaller numbing needle into the skin at the space between the two vertebrae. I injected slowly so as to allow the anesthetic to work on the skin pain receptors. Then I withdrew the needle and inserted the longer spinal needle. When it approached the spinal nerve, Joanne experienced a sensation of warmth and pain down her leg. I repositioned and checked that the tip of the needle was exactly where it should be, not too close and not too far from the fatty myelinated sheath of the spinal nerve.

I painted the spinal nerve on the fluoroscope screen using the clear contrast dye, which lit up into a black streak in the outline of the nerve root. The contrast flowed upstream into the spinal canal under the pedicle of the vertebra, flushing out the inflammatory cells and creating a pathway for the cocktail I was just mixing up. I drew up a potent mixture of anti-inflammatory steroids and local anesthetic and carefully bathed the nerve root and spinal disc with the pain-relieving mixture to decrease the pain and sensitivity of the compressed and inflamed nerve.

Patients often ask me what *exactly* is causing their pain. Answering this question is sometimes easy, other times anything but simple. For example, pain felt in the hip could be generated in the spine by a pinched nerve. Occasionally, we do a procedure and a patient will shout: "That's it! That's exactly where my pain is!" At that point, I know we've found the pain generator. The absence of pain afterward is another clear indicator that we're in the right place.

In Joanne's case, we got lucky. After the procedure, she felt complete pain relief, confirming the stenosis at that location as the pain generator. "That was easier than I expected," she said. It's not an uncommon response from patients who are fearful of having spinal injections. For many people, simply the thought of having a needle inserted into the spine is terrifying.

Naturally, patients wish they could just swallow a pill to get rid of the pain and the underlying problem. Oral medications can help and are usually tried before injections, but when a medication is taken orally, it has a long journey ahead of it before it can address the targeted pain. Upon entering your stomach, the pill is broken down into a more digestible form by natural acids. Then it's delivered to and broken down further by the liver before entering the bloodstream through the liver's circulatory system.

Once in the blood, the medication travels into the inferior vena cava, which empties into the heart's right atrium, the right ventricle, and into the pulmonary artery, where the drug is whisked to the lungs and then back to the left atrium via the pulmonary veins. Finally, the medication enters the aorta, the largest blood vessel in the human body. From there, it gets sent to the various organs of the body, including the brain, the kidneys, the spine, and so on, taking effect at various sites of action.

MAKING THE RIGHT DIAGNOSIS

In an older patient with low back pain, I might consider spinal stenosis or facet joint arthritis to be leading causes of pain. I might also try to rule out an abdominal aortic aneurysm, a kidney stone, or perhaps a tumor. Does the patient have a history of prostate or breast cancer? What other aspects of the patient's medical history might come into play? I also have to take other medical conditions into account. How might they interact with the treatment we want to administer?

If I suspect that inflammation is playing a role but the patient has a history of gastric ulcers or underlying kidney disease, non-steroidal anti-inflammatory drugs (NSAIDs) may not be a safe approach. However, opiate painkillers could cause the patient to become constipated. Constipation leads to straining, putting pressure on the spine, and that can cause excruciating pain or even worsen a disc herniation.

Ultimately, only a small portion of an oral dose will make it to the site of inflammation. While, of course, you could simply take a higher dosage of the drug, you are limited by the side effects of a particular drug and its unintended effects on the other organs getting exposed to it. By bypassing this oral route and injecting the steroids directly to the inflamed site, we deliver a higher dose to the site that actually needs the medication.

Despite their accuracy and strength, steroid anti-inflammatory drugs injected into the spine are not a guaranteed cure for spinal pain and inflammation. Generally, there are two factors that play a role in the transmission of pain down a spinal nerve. When pain travels down a nerve, we call this radiculitis or radiculopathy. (One of my frustrated patients said, "Radiculitis? How about: This is ridiculous!" Pain can clearly drive patients to a point of extreme frustration.)

When a disc herniates, it often compresses the spinal nerve, causing *mechanical* radiculitis around the nerve, which then causes *chemical* radiculitis. Steroids aren't great at treating the former, but they're pretty good at treating the latter. Rarely is one present without the other, though.

Joanne returned to my clinic a few weeks later. "I felt really good for four weeks," she told me. "Then the pain came back."

"If you are finding that there is daytime pain and discomfort," I said, "let's add in meloxicam, an anti-inflammatory like ibuprofen, to help you without making you sleepy or upsetting your stomach too much. I also think physical therapy would benefit you by giving you an improved range of motion. I want you to be more comfortable with your daily activities, without having to fear that the pain will limit you. Either way, we should also repeat the injection."

Typically, I explained, we try to repeat injections two or even three times and see if there is temporary or partial improvement; the effects may be additive. In some cases, the problem is reversible, as with acute disc herniations. The problem may fix itself about 80 percent of the time. In other cases, the problem is chronic but injections can help with symptom management or just occasional flare-ups. Some patients get months to years of relief after a spinal injection. Others, like Joanne, see only short-term relief.

"Aren't too many steroid shots bad for my body?" she asked.

"Steroids are naturally occurring substances produced by the adrenal gland," I explained. "They help regulate many processes in our body. Getting a dose from an outside source just leads the body to produce a little less to balance things out. If you get too much from external sources, one complication is adrenal suppression: the adrenal gland shuts down and simply stops producing steroids, which can have negative consequences. Fortunately, adrenal suppression is exceedingly rare."

Some studies suggest that there is a benefit to injecting local anesthetic alone in the spine. In these cases, it may be that numbing the pain tricks the nervous system so it stops signaling for inflammatory cells to aggregate in a particular area. This can reduce inflammation.

Perhaps we are simply rinsing away the inflammatory cells and helping to rewire the body's neurological pathways through neuroplasticity. The washing away of inflammatory cells would be similar to the incision and drainage we perform on certain infections that have formed a pus pocket, using saline or antibiotic fluid to wash away any bacteria and help the body rid itself of the bacterial invaders. As we discussed earlier, the sensory and immune systems work together, in a coordinated fashion, to respond to a site where pain or inflammation has occurred.

In Joanne's case, we repeated the injection and, again, only a few weeks of relief occurred before the pain returned. This was a classic case of mechanical radiculitis as the underlying problem, with chemical radiculitis on top of it. In other words, the nerve was getting rubbed and scuffed up in a tight space. We weren't treating the mechanical damage, only the resulting inflammation.

The real problem was the stenosis, the narrowing at the foramen where the nerve exited the spine, resulting in painful compression. Joanne had scoliosis in that part of her spine and, unless a minimally invasive surgery to widen the foramen could be performed, a spinal fusion might become necessary.

Luckily, the spine surgeon successfully managed the foraminal widening procedure, and ultimately Joanne had complete relief of her pain symptoms without a major surgery to correct her scoliosis.

A spine-surgical colleague, Jay Khanna at Johns Hopkins, told me, "Of all the non-operative things I prescribe to my patients with spinal stenosis, the one that helps them the most is spinal injections in pain management. Although the literature says that such injections don't change the underlying problem, I think that injections allow for very effective pain control and symptom management for the short-term and sometimes the long-term, while the body heals itself naturally. If I didn't refer out as many of my patients for pain management, I would operate about twice as much as I do now."

I recently spoke to Joanne and asked her about her experience. She was quite happy to be feeling better and to have avoided a spinal fusion. Upon reflection, her experience with pain was a dark period in her life. "I didn't know how severe pain could be until I had nerve pain. Nerve pain is worse than childbirth. I've had experiences with pain and thought I was pretty tough because of those, but nerve pain is just a whole different level of pain. I now have breast cancer and all the treatments I am going through are a walk in the park compared to the spinal pain I experienced."

I was shocked at this statement, but also intrigued. Could pain somehow make a person stronger?

HOW SOON DO I GET RELIEF?

"So when am I going to feel better?"

I get this question a lot. It speaks to the urgency people feel when they are experiencing pain. Pain takes priority. Fortunately, there are several options for pain management.

Epidural injections are quite common in managing spinal pain. There are two types: *interlaminar* or *transforaminal* (the latter is also called a selective nerve root injection). The major difference is how the needle is placed in the spine. The objective is the same: to deliver a targeted dose of medication to the area where the pain is coming from.

Although we view these injections as less risky than surgery, there is controversy as to whether they are truly effective in the long-term. In the short-term, there is a clear benefit to spinal injections. We frequently inject steroids and local anesthetic into areas of inflammation to provide pain relief. In these instances, I explain that steroids take up to 10 days to become effective, though people often feel better right away from the local anesthetic.

"Can I only get three shots of cortisone in my lifetime?" patients often ask.

"No, more like three in a six-month period, up to a maximum of four to six injections in a year," I explain. We find that initially patients need this number of injections because, in some cases, we are still trying to establish the diagnosis of the "pain generator." Once the pain generator has been found and treated, the frequency of steroid injections is reduced. There are also many steroid-free treatments we can offer, such as spinal cord stimulation and radiofrequency ablation for painful nerves. Patients that don't respond to steroids or have already been treated with the maximum amount still have other options for pain management. In some cases, where steroids are contraindicated, we may use local anesthetics to help with pain.

Just like anything in life, too much of a good thing can be harmful, and steroids are no exception. Rheumatologists, who specialize in treating inflammatory disorders, often inject steroids into arthritic joints. Steroids are also used orally to treat chronic conditions such as rheumatoid arthritis. But too many steroids can cause problems such as osteoporosis, adrenal suppression, and poor wound healing because they can inhibit collagen formation and osteoblast activity. We have to strike a balance between these risks and benefits.

When I bring up steroids, patients often think of *anabolic steroids*, like the type bodybuilders use. "Doc, am I gonna look like the Hulk tomorrow?" they ask. The steroids used in pain management aren't those types of steroids. These are steroids that decrease inflammation as opposed to adding muscle bulk.

Roughly 1 in 10 patients with neck pain and/or radiating arm pain will need surgery. From a pain management perspective, we try to exhaust the conservative options first before proceeding with surgery. When surgery is necessary, if the pain generator is clearly defined, surgical outcomes are likely to be better. Along the way, we usually have input from and work closely with spine surgeons to figure this out.

I remember when one of my attending physicians during my fellowship at Brigham and Women's Hospital told a frustrated patient with chronic pain, "We're called *pain management, not pain solutions.*"

"I wish I had something else to offer you," I say when it seems that surgery is a patient's only remaining option. At least then, patients can go into surgery confident that they've tried every available option from a conservative therapy standpoint.

When I perform injections, I am usually introducing a needle into an already painful area. Most of the time when physicians administer injections, or introduce needles through the skin (e.g., as in acupuncture), the site of the shot is not already painful. For example, flu shots are injected into healthy, pain-free tissue. This is not the case in shots to reduce pain. As a result, "How much is it gonna hurt?" is always a tough question for me to answer.

Patients are understandably nervous about being stuck with a needle in a site that is already painful. There are so many factors in this situation. For example, the pain threshold and pain tolerance of the individual patient both play a role. *Pain threshold* is defined as the degree of stimulus that is felt as pain. *Pain tolerance* is the point at which a patient can no longer tolerate the pain. Both of these are important factors, but we don't have an easy way of measuring them in practice, as we do in a research laboratory.

Anxiety about the procedure plays a major role in how a patient will perceive the pain and how much they can tolerate during the injection. The amount of inflammation present, the level of wind-up, and a person's hyper-responsiveness to pain, also influence how much pain a person will experience during a procedure. This physical reaction plays a role because I will often get close to the nerve without quite touching it. Often patients will report shooting pain in a leg before I am truly in contact with the nerve root, likely from the sensitization of other nerves in the vicinity. We also know genetics can play a role in pain threshold and tolerance.

Unfortunately, injecting local anesthesia alone will not make the area completely numb. In many cases, it will actually burn as it's introduced, which will drive up fear and anxiety when the longer spinal needle is inserted. This scenario clearly shows how pain is eventually interpreted in the brain. Individuals react differently to the same stimulus, in this case, a needle penetrating the skin. Some people are perfectly still and calm, hardly flinching during the procedure. Others move reflexively as the needle advances millimeter by millimeter, even through anesthetized tissue. Sometimes, a patient will jerk away upon injection of the local anesthetic.

It is this exact variability that makes pain studies hard. You could even say that this variability is a hallmark of pain, which is why managing pain is as much of an art as a science.

IMAGING THE PAINFUL SPINE

Imaging the spine with an MRI can be very helpful in this regard. Some physicians treat clinically, based on the pain pattern (der-matome) or the area of muscle pain or weakness (myotome). I have found this information misleading at times, because it leads doctors to act on an assumption.

My practice in most cases is to order an MRI prior to the injection. This strategy minimizes the variability of the response and allows for better targeting of the steroid to the inflammatory source in the spine. Sometimes, however, insurance companies don't approve MRI imaging. In this era of controlling health care costs, it can be difficult to get one authorized. I know that we will have problems when my assistant tells me that the insurance company wants to do a *peer-to-peer review*. I reluctantly get on the phone with them, often getting put on hold while the patient sees their scheduled appointment time slip by.

"Dr. Singla," they'll say, "our guidelines state that your patient has to have six weeks of conservative therapy before an MRI."

"Yes," I reply, "but this patient is in significant pain and I want the MRI so it can help guide the next steps in therapy. We've tried medication and physical therapy already."

"I understand, but our guidelines state...."

It's frustrating. When we don't have proper imaging to care for our spinal pain patients, the following things tend to happen:

- We end up spending money on more injections to get the patient a therapeutic effect. This happens because you are initially guessing where the disc herniation or other spinal pain generator is located by trial and error.

- There is attribution bias leading you away from the true pain generator. For example, if a doctor believes it's a disc herniation but it's actually piriformis syndrome compressing the sciatic nerve, time and money will be wasted pursuing the improper treatment. A lumbar MRI could rule out disc herniation early, to direct the physician to treat the actual cause.

- More opiate medications are prescribed to treat the patient's pain while the doctor seeks a definitive diagnosis. This increases opiate-related issues as discussed in Chapter 5.

- Patients miss more time from work and continue to experience heightened levels of pain. Anxiety increases as time passes and doctors have difficulty finding the true pain generator.

- Patients suffer from more physical deconditioning due to a lack of activity. Patients worry about making the pain or injury worse, so they stop doing anything that they think could result in structural damage.

It's an understatement to say that insurance companies and the medical system in general fail to understand the psychological impact of pain and its impact on a person's life. The medical system understands acute injury or any easily identifiable condition that can be quantified and treated. But when patients are in our office, suffering, doctors need the proper tools to diagnose and treat pain. Instead, the health care system often erects more barriers to appropriate and effective care.

With professional athletes, an MRI is often obtained immediately after a suspected injury. Team physicians quickly find out how long their athletes will be on the sidelines, and an appropriate plan is made for treatment. When a regular person's physician requests imaging, I believe, similar urgency and priority should be granted, provided that the imaging request is relevant to the presenting problem.

What is unfortunate about this trend is that early MRIs and other imaging often reduce costs to the health care system (and to society), especially in cases where a patient's pain lasts more than a few weeks. Doctors can utilize it appropriately to pinpoint pain generators and aggressively treat them. I am by no means advocating that we get MRIs of the spines of everyone who has brief, mild, or self-limited pain that improves within days or weeks. As a pain specialist, I see the tougher cases. Therefore, when I order an MRI, patients have already been through the gauntlet of treatment because their pain symptoms have not improved for a significant period of time or with the usual interventions.

I recall a recent insurance company peer-to-peer conversation regarding an 80-year-old patient with low back pain. The physician on the other line was a spine surgeon. I breathed a sigh of relief, figuring he would be sympathetic to my predicament and let me order a lumbar MRI. After all, he understood the spine and its pain generators. Instead, his response was negative.

"But we need some help here," I said. "I think the patient has a disc herniation." I needed to pinpoint the level of the herniation so I could deliver an epidural steroid injection to the proper level in his spine.

"Dr. Singla," he said, "this patient is 80. I've never seen a disc herniation in an 80-year-old. It's probably just spinal stenosis."

"I respectfully disagree," I replied. "I have seen disc herniations in patients this age."

"We're just going to have to agree to disagree here," he said. "I'm denying the MRI."

If your practice doesn't order MRIs for patients this age, I wondered to myself, how would you ever know it *wasn't* a disc herniation? You don't know what you're missing if you don't order the test. Less than a week later, I saw a disc extrusion—the most advanced type of disc herniation—in a 90-year-old patient after her MRI.

"Why don't you just do an epidural steroid injection and see what happens?"

And what if it wasn't a disc herniation? One to three percent of the time, it's an uncommon cause such as a tumor, aneurysm, or infection. The imaging helps us rule out these less common causes of pain.

I really do believe that the injection (with or without steroids) has to go right to the source of inflammation in order to be the most effective. This is based on both empirical evidence and my own professional experience. The risk of not performing these injections is that there will be persistent inflammation, possible nerve injury, and subsequent wind-up with far worse pain.

I recall a case where the patient had an acute L2-3 disc herniation. Although my practice is to inject the medication at the site of the pain generator, he had seen another pain physician who had performed an epidural steroid injection at L5-S1. The patient didn't feel better and subsequently came to see me. I reviewed the information and decided to opt for a second injection directly at the L2-3 level. He experienced complete relief and didn't have any further symptoms after the injection.

What is the risk of injecting the spine without a prior MRI? If a patient improves with the injection, it is likely that the MRI will not be ordered or completed. In this scenario, you potentially miss problems like tumors or infections that are not ordinary mechanical spine issues. This is another reason I like to obtain an MRI, to better pinpoint the structural spine problem if one exists and to rule out a serious problem.

The data is conflicting regarding spinal injections. To debate the pros and cons based on the literature would be beyond the scope of this book. I think most physicians agree that:

1. There is likely significant short-term benefit from epidural steroid injections to treat disc herniations or spinal stenosis, and possible long-term benefits as well.

2. Although catastrophic complications are rare, injections are less risky and less expensive than spinal surgery and may help some people avoid surgery.

3. The risk of catastrophic complications is rare, and therefore injections are worth considering in patients who fail conscrvative therapy with medications and physical therapy. They are especially worth considering when function is limited, or when moderate to severe pain is present.

Would some patients get better without injections? Maybe. But, based on my observations, it would likely take longer and result in missed work or decreased functioning.

Good-quality studies vary on the benefits of epidural steroids for spinal pain. The evidence does point to short-term benefit addressing radiating pain in the leg or arm.

I'd like to comment here on research studies. Randomized, controlled trials (RCTs) are helpful in establishing a high standard of science in our lives, but at the end of the day, the body is a complex system with many inputs and interactions producing the final outcome. We still have much to learn about the human body, its genetics, receptors, and physiology. When studying a certain aspect of the body or a drug in isolation, we may miss an undiscovered therapeutic opportunity if the study fails to demonstrate benefits in a particular scenario. This may in part be due to the limitations of the study. The doctors that do rely exclusively on science may have suboptimal outcomes if the art of medicine is totally ignored.

Meanwhile, insurance companies look at these randomized studies (or lack thereof) as a great opportunity to deny payment for treatments. This methodology ignores the fact that the treatment may have been helpful in a subset of thc population or, as is the case with epidural steroid injections, these may help avoid a more expensive or risky intervention such as surgery. By treating symptoms without understanding the disease process, you may miss the bigger picture.

Ray Kurzweil, in his book *How to Create a Mind,* states that "the world of art is actually ahead of the world of science in appreciating the power of the human perceptual system." Art is about pattern recognition. There are subtle patterns of perception that guide us as physicians in how we treat patients. Sometimes, it's not so apparent to an outside observer, but they involve how we organize information and the connections we have established in our brains.

A well-cited article in the *British Medical Journal* makes an important point about the power of observation:

As with many interventions intended to prevent ill health, the effectiveness of parachutes [to prevent major trauma when jumping from an airplane] has not been subjected to rigorous evaluation by using randomised controlled trials. Advocates of evidence-based medicine have criticised the adoption of interventions evaluated by using only observational data. We think that everyone might benefit if the most radical protagonists of evidence-based medicine organised and participated in a double-blind, randomised, placebo-controlled, crossover trial of the parachute.

This is dry British humor at its best. Of course, no one is going to jump out of an airplane without a parachute to help prove that parachutes work. Certain interventions in medicine, through observation appear to work. When health insurance companies deny care based on a philosophy of "evidence-based medicine," they are often simply denying care to save money in the interest of the bottom line.

David Caraway is a well-known pain specialist. He states:

Chronic pain is a complex process with many inputs into the system. The effect of one therapy on a specific patient can be quite variable due to individual differences. While well-designed randomized, double-blind, controlled trials may demonstrate benefit for the study population, they do not guarantee a similar response in all patients. Also, some treatments that don't have RCTs may in fact provide benefit in certain individuals. An insurance company may develop their own criteria for judging evidence, and in many cases they may use their rules rather than the physician's clinical judgment, often denying payment for effective treatments.

In his book *How Doctors Think*, Jerome Groopman makes the same comment regarding evidence-based medicine: "Statistics cannot substitute for the human being before you; numbers can only complement a physician's personal experience with a drug or procedure."

So, if you tell a patient there is a 62 percent chance they have a disease, what does that mean to the patient? Either they have the disease (100 percent) or they don't (0 percent). Statistics don't help you identify the specific problem in the patient sitting in front of you.

FINDING THE PAIN GENERATOR

Most (95 percent) of lumbar disc herniations occur at the bottom two levels of the spine, at L4-5 and L5-S1. This is not surprising, given that they bear the most load. The nerves at these levels are closely intertwined with the fixed, bony sacrum and the pelvis. They bear the brunt of the motion stresses with bending, lifting, and twisting. When a patient has a disc herniation, I generally advise "no BLTs."

When we make a decision to perform injections, we try to target the pain generator to decrease the pain and the inflammation. However, I'm careful to inform my patients that there is usually some trial and error involved.

If there is residual pain, we look at secondary targets such as the lumbar facet joints or the sacroiliac joints. If the pain is muscular, or myofascial, we can perform trigger point injections. Physical therapy is necessary if function is compromised, or if patients are fearful of doing something that might exacerbate the pain. A multimodal strategy for pain management is important.

"After the shots," patients ask, "am I going to know if I'm doing something to damage my body?"

"Luckily," I reply, "the body is intelligent enough to still deliver the damage warning signal to you despite my best efforts to shut it down and decrease it."

After conservative therapy, if the pain persists or there is evidence of a neurologic deficit (such as weakness or numbness), I send patients to see a spine surgeon. There are two types of spine surgeons: neurosurgeons and orthopedic surgeons. Both have residency training in their surgical specialty, and many pursue fellowship training above and beyond that in spine surgery.

While the evidence is debated, I observe relief from injections in well above half my patients, generally for several weeks or even months. If the problem is one that can improve on its own, like a new disc herniation, it will likely get better without surgery unless there is serious nerve root compression or stenosis.

ALTERNATIVE TREATMENTS FOR CHRONIC PAIN

I often get questions about whether my patients should pursue acupuncture for their pain management. In the past, I've told them that I didn't know much about it. Finally, I made it a point to find out. I called up David Euler, an instructor in Harvard Medical School's acupuncture course for physicians.

Euler, a fit, worldly man in his mid-50s with sandy brown hair and infectious enthusiasm, sat down with me over a drink one afternoon. Originally from Germany but having grown up in Israel, Euler was a rescue-and-extraction paramedic in the Israeli army and subsequently went to medical school.

In military service, he often found himself dealing with life-and-death scenarios. Euler found the work rewarding. It was almost always clear what needed to be done. Regarding wounded soldiers, he remarked "It's pretty clear they need oxygen when their face is blue," Euler explained. "Then you get an airway, either through intubation or a tracheotomy. Suddenly, they're pink again, and alive."

We turned to the topic of acupuncture, and why he pursued it.

"After my experience in the military," he told me, "I wanted to try something a bit different from traditional medicine. What interested me about acupuncture was that it takes a whole-body approach that has not changed much in over two thousand years. There's some sustaining truth and wisdom behind that. With medicine, things are changing so much that we often go down a path and ten years later realize what we did was wrong, as happened with opiates for chronic pain."

Euler isn't certain how acupuncture helps with pain. He has theories, though. According to him, there are likely three things it does for patients in pain:

- Fascial tissue planes loosen and relax, which may help with referred pain.

- Acupuncture has a calming psychological impact that affects the perception of physical pain.

- It helps restore balance between the sympathetic and parasympathetic nervous system.

In other words, it helps get the body out of fight-or-flight mode.

"Sometimes with pain," Euler told me, "it's simply a matter of validation that the patient is suffering."

Another alternative therapy is mindfulness meditation. A recent article in the *Journal of Neuroscience* showed that mindfulness meditation reduced pain more effectively than placebo methods. The researchers used fMRI to show which specific regions of the brain became activated during meditation. Structures known to be involved in chronic pain from other fMRI studies were among those activated. There are conflicting studies as to whether meditation involves endogenous opiate release and effects.

Other treatments we use for chronic pain include yoga, physical therapy, chiropractic therapy, hypnosis, exercise, stretching, tai chi, and cognitive-behavioral therapy.

Barriers to more widespread adoption of these non-traditional treatment options do exist, primarily on the side of insurance companies. Hopefully, with a shift to a more value-based health care system in the United States, these therapies will become more available as alternatives to opiate therapy or when traditional therapy fails.

ANOTHER PERSONAL EXPERIENCE WITH PAIN

Two years ago, I began experiencing neck pain, which progressively worsened. Interventional pain physicians wear lead around our necks to protect our thyroid gland from the harmful effects of ionizing radiation. The fluoroscope, which we use to deliver our injections in a precise manner, does emit radiation, so we have to make sure we are protected. Over time, however, this added weight, along with bending, turning, and twisting can cause structural injury to the tissues of the neck and cervical spine.

I went to see Mayo Friedlis, a colleague and fellow pain physician. I had already tried trigger point injections, topical patches, and NSAIDs along with traction and physical therapy. Friedlis reviewed my cervical MRI, which was essentially normal. On flexion and extension films, he saw what is known as subluxation, or movement between the vertebrae in my neck from a flexed versus an extended position.

This kind of instability is thought to be one cause of neck and back pain. In fact, joint instability from loose ligaments is considered one of the main causes of joint pain in our bodies. As we get older, ligaments get lax, tendons and muscles and other soft tissues stretch and elongate, and stability is reduced around the joints in our body. The joint surfaces start to slide against one another, resulting in friction and inflammation. This is probably a very early symptom of the development of joint arthritis. There's a good chance that the bending and turning I was doing with the lead collar had taken its toll on my neck ligaments.

I did some research on ligamentous laxity and found that, although there is fairly good evidence that this is a contributing factor to development of osteoarthritis of the knee, there wasn't much evidence regarding the spine.

"There is a newer option available," Friedlis told me. "It's called regenerative therapy. We take some of your blood, spin it down to get the nutrients out, and then inject that into the site where your spine is moving to tighten up and regenerate the ligaments. It'll reduce your pain, and more importantly, reduce the motion in your spine by treating your underlying problem instead of just the symptoms."

Sounds good, I thought, but will it work? Regenerative therapy was still considered experimental because the results had not been scrutinized in large, controlled trials. I scoured the literature and looked for as much high-quality data as I could find. Platelet-rich plasma (PRP), the substance injected at the site of the injury, had been used by high-profile athletes like Kobe Bryant and Tiger Woods. It appeared to stimulate healing by delivering a high concentration of cell nutrients and growth factors to an area of injury.

Friedlis performed three sessions of injections into the cervical spine. Over time, I felt less laxity in the ligaments and a significant reduction in pain.

Most recently, Stephen Curry of the Golden State Warriors was diagnosed with a medial collateral ligament (MCL) strain before the NBA playoffs in 2016. His doctors tried regenerative therapy on the injury and he went on to compete in the finals. He may have felt better, but Cleveland still won a historic seven-game series against the Warriors.

Today, some physicians employ stem cells to help with tissue regeneration and to treat spinal pain by helping to regrow damaged tissue. Again, there are not a lot of high-quality studies, only early experimental data, but it may be a promising avenue of treatment.

Futurist Ray Kurzweil says that one day in the near future, we are all going to be like cars—regenerating tissue and organs to replace damaged parts. "Theoretically," he says, "we can run a car forever. You just have to keep changing parts." That's a discussion for another day—but maybe sooner than we think. As for today, we are just scratching the surface with regards to treatments for pain, especially those that address the underlying problem as opposed to simply managing the painful symptoms. The future holds promising options for treatment of the underlying problems as well as newer and more effective ways of managing the symptoms of pain.

CHAPTER 8

THE ONLY EASY DAY WAS YESTERDAY

> Hardship can create a helpless person or a heroic one.
> Some people are made stronger by suffering. Others
> are defeated. The difference is resilience.
>
> —ERIC GREITENS, *Resilience*

"EVERYTHING HAPPENS FOR A REASON" was the inscription on Ellen's wrist bracelet. For some reason, my attention was drawn to it as I went over the young woman's MRI results with her.

"It hurts here," she said, gesturing to her spine, right below the bra strap.

"Can you bend?" I asked.

"Yes." With difficulty, I could see. "I slipped on the steps and hit my back pretty hard."

"You have a compression fracture of the T10 vertebrae," I told her, looking at the MRI. "It probably happened when you slipped and fell."

Vertebral compression fractures (VCFs) of the spine are increasing in the United States and other places with aging populations. Aging leads to a process in our bones known as *osteopenia* or, in its more severe form, *osteoporosis*. Basically, more bone is taken away than is rebuilt. Our bodies are building bone until the age of 25 or so, then things start to go in the other direction.

We talked through the options. Ellen was a teacher. She would have to take the rest of the school year off. She could not stand or bend due to the pain from the injury. She wore a brace and, although that alleviated the pain, it was causing pressure on other areas and restricting her motion.

"I'm just ready to get this thing taken care of," Ellen told me. "I don't want to keep trying Band-Aid [solutions]."

We decided that if she didn't feel better three months after the fracture—VCFs can heal on their own—we were going to perform a *kyphoplasty*, injecting special cement into the spinal bones to strengthen them, stop the pain, and prevent further collapse in height. Three months went by and Ellen returned to my office in pain. It was clear we'd need to do the procedure.

We positioned Ellen on her belly and gave some antibiotics through her intravenous line. After numbing up the skin, I went into the spinal bone with a needle, through the pedicle, the round strut that connects the front and rear of the spinal bone like the chassis of a car.

Once inside the spinal bone, I inflated a balloon to create some space and then filled up that space with a dough-like cement material, which would harden into an area as strong as healthy bone. I withdrew the needle, closed the incision with sterile adhesive strips, and put on a clean dressing. Ten minutes later, the cement had set and Ellen was able to get up. No pain, a good early sign.

Soon after, Ellen was out of the brace. She was ready to get back to her life. I told her we weren't quite done yet. Even though the VCF was a result of an injury, we needed to know if she was starting to develop thinning of the bones, which may have contributed to the fracture. I ordered a bone density scan. It revealed that, despite her young age, Ellen had early-onset osteoporosis, putting her at risk for more fractures.

"Remember the inscription on your bracelet?" I said. "Well, if we say anything good might have come out of this, it's that we figured out why you had the fracture. Your bones are thinner than we would expect. Luckily, we have a treatment for you to prevent more of these." I sent her to a rheumatologist who agreed to start her on a bone-building drug to significantly reduce her risk of spinal fractures down the road.

"I guess I'm thankful we figured this out early," Ellen told me. "Maybe there is something good that came out of my pain."

DEFINING RESILIENCE

What is the real meaning and purpose of pain?

I'm not a philosopher, but this is still a question I get asked by patients all the time. Eventually, I decided I may as well try to have some sort of answer rather than look at them blankly.

I decided to pick up some books, look online, and speak to some colleagues and friends about the deeper meaning of pain and suffering. As physicians, we're taught about alleviating suffering, and about developing compassion and empathy for our patients. But is there a purpose to suffering? I wasn't so sure. Sure, pain can be a turning point and it can help us grow. But *why?* The answer wasn't nearly as easy to spot as a broken vertebra on an X-ray.

Life is a struggle for survival that begins at conception.

Millions of sperm fight their way to the egg to fertilize it. Only the strongest, fastest, most qualified one makes it. And the competition is only just beginning.

How do we rise to the challenge of pain? We can't cheat it without consequences. The only approach that makes sense is one of resilience, to use the experience of pain to help us better cope with adversity. I'm by no means wishing pain on anyone. Rather, I'm saying that the only possible way to live a full life is to face pain head-on, transforming it into something that leaves you better equipped to face life's challenges.

I spoke with Alan Sheff, a primary-care physician in Maryland. We've worked together on several patient cases. Sheff, an insightful and thorough physician, had some thoughts to share.

"Pain is definitely an alarm," he told me, "but patients are so focused on the pain that they forget the underlying reason for it." Sheff had hip arthritis. It became so severe that he had difficulty with daily functioning. Eventually, he went in to have a hip joint replacement surgery. "When my patients ask me when to have surgery for a problem, I tell them, when you find it hard to do basic things like drive a car, sit in a chair, or walk the dog. Then it's time."

Sheff continued to struggle with pain after his hip replacement surgery.

"I had this persistent pain and inflammation that lasted a long time," he said. "It would sometimes come out of nowhere and just grab me. One day, I was walking outside and I had this sudden severe bout of pain. I stopped, looked around. I saw the sun shining, I could hear the birds chirping, and realized that maybe I just needed to slow down and enjoy life a bit more. The longer it took me to walk to my car, the more I could appreciate what was around me. Pain made me stop and realize that there was more to life than working and rushing around. So I gave my pain a name: Patience. It was there to teach me that I needed to step back and enjoy life a bit more."

How do we learn to better cope with pain? No one really teaches us this growing up. Can you imagine a high school class called "Dealing with your pain"?

Pain is something we learn to deal with in our own way. Whether we name it, compartmentalize it, or distract ourselves from it, there's no better teacher than experience. Sure, some coping methods are better than others, and we have tools to manage or treat pain, but I believe coping through resilience to some degree is an adaptive quality that we all can and should learn.

The inability to cope with life's stresses results in maladaptive coping behaviors. As you already know from earlier chapters, the emotional response to pain can significantly amplify or limit the pain experience. Resilience is how we meet with adversity and pain. In order to survive, we need be able to process negative experiences into positive growth.

How does one become resilient? Is it something we're born with, or something we learn in life? It turns out to be a bit of both. In a recent article in *British Journal of Psychology*, a longitudinal study of 7,500 twins revealed that psychological resilience is approximately 50 percent genetic and 50 percent environmental. Nature and nurture are both equally important in the process.

In speaking with several physicians in different fields, I've found that most agree with this based on their own observations. Research shows there are clearly genes that regulate pain and that genetic variations can render a person more or less susceptible to it. Are there genes that produce adaptive resilience?

This is the classic nature-versus-nurture argument. I believe that humans develop resilience by stimulating the nervous system to process adverse experiences or painful stimuli and forcing ourselves to survive or overcome these circumstances. A graphical representation of how I view resilience, based on the classic definition of "toughness, or the ability to adjust to misfortune or change" is *function* on the y-axis, in the setting of *pain*, on the x-axis. It looks something like this:

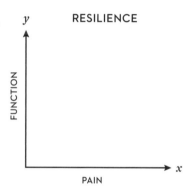

Next, take a look at what high and low resilience, respectively, might look like:

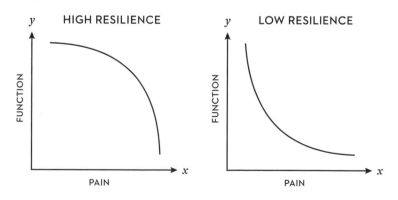

A high-resilience person would keep functioning reasonably well despite pain. A low-resilience person would, at the very early occurrence of pain, see a drop-off in function. Resilience is a trait that can be improved over time. Patients tell me that pain focuses them in a way unlike other experiences. Pain is urgent. It forces you into action. You must find a way to manage it or it will manage you. It can restore purpose to your life if you can find meaning in the suffering.

Is the purpose of pain to not only alert us, but to also somehow awaken us? Is pain a mechanism through which we can become more resilient? Among those who have survived a painful experience, none want to repeat the experience, but most believe they are wiser as a result of it.

THE HEART RISES TO THE OCCASION

Earlier we talked about takotsubo syndrome (i.e., broken heart syndrome), where overwhelming mental, and sometimes physical, stress causes one to have a severe weakening of the heart muscle, which feels almost exactly like a heart attack. On imaging, the heart swells up like a balloon and diagnostic tests will indicate a heart attack.

This is a real condition, though rare. If you look closely at the physiology of the heart, you will see that it actually evolved to rise to the challenge when stressed. The difference between the two outcomes appears to be in what your mind tells it to do. Your heart is basically a pump to send blood to our organs. During periods of increased oxygen demand—exercise, illness, stress—the heart is designed to work harder.

Frank Starling came up with what are now known as Starling

curves to show how the heart reacts when the brain calls on it to pump more oxygen to our tissues, and looks like this:

STARLING CURVES FOR HEART

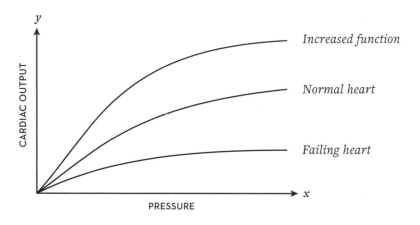

Cardiac output (CO) is how much blood and oxygen the heart can pump in a certain amount of time. Your heart rate (HR) multiplied by your Stroke Volume (SV), how much blood is in one squeeze of the heart, determines how much oxygen you can pump into your tissues:

$$CO = HR \times SV$$

Notice how, on the Starling curves, as pressure in the normal heart increases, output should increase as well. Many naturally gifted athletes have low resting heart rates, 40 to 60 beats per minute. This allows them to increase the amount of oxygen delivery to their bodies (and hence, output) and push themselves further than someone with a more typical resting heart rate of 78. In other words, they have more natural reserve.

This doesn't mean a person with a higher resting heart rate can't train for a marathon or compete in the Olympics. It might take more work in the mental arena, more training, but the adaptive nature of our bodies can compensate for a genetic disadvantage.

We don't quite have the machinery to look inside the head and define psychological resilience, however, we do have the ability to look at real-life examples and extrapolate from them, using the heart as a basic model of how the human body was designed to rise to the challenge.

If our basic biology is inherently programmed to rise to the challenge and meet the demands placed on it, then how should we extrapolate this to our own selves in the face of adversity? I believe we all must rise to the occasion when facing adversity, as the heart increases the supply of oxygen to our organs. The heart continues its life-sustaining purpose by delivering oxygen when we are stressed. When we experience pain, whether physical or psychological, we must gather our mental strength and meet the pain head on. Floundering in the face of adversity is not something we can afford individually or collectively.

THE BRITISH INVASION IN WORLD WAR II

In *David and Goliath*, Malcolm Gladwell discusses an excellent example of resilience in the British response to the Blitz, the unceasing bombing of London by the Germans during World War II:

On the eve of the war, in 1937, the British military issued a dire prediction that German bombing would result in 600,000 casualties and 1.2 million wounded in London.

Mass panic was predicted, and a halt in industrial production was forecast because people would not go to work, instead staying home or in bomb shelters. The military predicted that if this happened, they would likely lose the war.

In 1940 when the attack began, the exact opposite occurred. Despite tens of thousands of bombs and a million incendiary devices resulting in 40,000 deaths and 46,000 injuries, mass panic never came. People continued on as if nothing was happening, despite shrapnel and flames everywhere.

Psychiatrist J. T. MacCurdy, according to Gladwell, came up with an explanation. He divided Londoners into three groups. Group 1 was those killed by the bombs. Group 2 was those "near-misses" who were in shock but still alive. Group 3 were "remote misses"—the majority of the population—who could see what was happening but self-identified as survivors. This emboldens Group 3, providing them with excitement and a sense of invulnerability. (Remember, with 8 million people in London, only a small minority were harmed by the bombs.)

When a bomb missed a citizen in London, they would continue on as if they could not be harmed. They would actually go outside more and do more. You could imagine them saying, "If I haven't been hit yet, maybe it's not meant to happen." The same was seen in several other countries where civilians were unexpectedly resilient in the face of bombing.

To me, this is a classic example of resilience. As physicians, we could learn some lessons from this to continue to try very hard to encourage our patients to stay functional in the setting of pain.

Earlier, when I discussed Jim, the case with phantom pain, he demonstrated remarkable resilience. After this experience, and when we discussed his amputation pain and the life impact of his phantom pain, he said that "God gives us what we can handle."

This is a Biblical statement I have never forgotten—even more so considering it came from someone missing a limb and in pain exactly where he had no limb present. But it also points to how some people use religious beliefs to cope with adversity and build the resilience necessary to tackle life's challenges.

In his book *Long Walk to Freedom*, Nelson Mandela wrote: "To be truly prepared for something, one must actually expect it. One cannot be prepared for something while secretly believing it will not happen. We were all prepared (for death) not because we were brave, but because we were realistic." I think this has applications to pain as well and our expectations around it.

AN EXAMPLE OF RESILIENCE

Brian was by all measures a successful individual. In the Air Force Special Forces, he served with honor in military conflicts. For Brian, jumping out of helicopters and planes was actually fun, satisfying his craving for adventure.

After leaving the military, Brian became a police officer and took up hunting and fishing as hobbies. A gifted athlete, Brian also became a powerlifter, maxing out at a full 635 pounds on the bench press. He also competed in strong man competitions, once pulling a fire truck by himself.

Brian was no stranger to pain. After his usual workout routine of completing 500 reps of a 135-pound bench press, his shoulders were burning, but he forced himself to ignore the pain, and it usually went away. Another painful experience came the day he saw a car on a collision path with his son. He sprang into action, barely noticing a loud snap, like a gunshot, as he raced over and pulled the boy out of harm's way. No one was hit by the car, but Brian discovered that he had snapped the plantar fascia in his foot, which brought incredible pain once he had a moment to let his adrenaline settle down.

Despite these intensely painful incidents, nothing could prepare him for what he experienced in the spring of 2014. On a sunny and clear day, Brian was practicing his golf game at the range. He bent over to pick up a ball to place on the tee and felt a sudden, electrical jolt of pain into his left buttock and groin. He decided to stop playing for a bit and see if this would resolve on its own. But it didn't go away. It got worse.

Brian eventually had to call an ambulance when the pain got so bad he dropped to the floor. He was given 20 milligrams of intravenous morphine, which didn't put a dent in the pain, so he was taken to the emergency room. Only after multiple, high doses of narcotics did his pain come under control. Now, I had to figure out what had caused it.

What eventually led to our diagnosis was his lumbar MRI, which showed compression of his left L5 nerve root. An injection reproduced his pain but gave little lasting relief, so we surmised that it was mechanical compression, not simply inflammation around the nerve, causing this unremitting pain.

I sent Brian to a spine surgeon. The surgeon was initially reluctant to operate, but given the data, we felt pretty good about the pain being limited to L5-S1.

During surgery, the spine surgeon noticed that the L5 nerve root was crushed between the unstable L5 and S1 vertebrae. He decompressed the nerve and performed a spinal fusion, where two spinal bones are put together as a single, solid block held together by rods and screws, like two square blocks clamped and held together so they can't perform a motion that might pinch the nerve again.

The severe pain improved. Brian said the nerve pain was worse than any other pain that he had experienced before. He was hesitant, but started slowly to resume his activities.

Talking to me, Brian reflected on his father's passing away suddenly while he was still young, and how it had impacted him and his family. While Brian was no slouch previously, health took on a new meaning for him. I advised him to take up swimming, to limit the stress of gravity on his body as he was healing. He began swimming regularly.

One year after surgery, Brian had dropped from 310 lbs. to 235 lbs., fitter than ever. He was back to playing golf, biking, and his other normal activities. He was in many ways changed by the pain, but he was better off in terms of his overall health and his level of fitness. He was better for having gone through this painful experience in his life.

"Pain was a turning point for me."

* * *

I recently spoke with Dan Valaik, an orthopedic surgeon with John Hopkins. "Clearly pain can be debilitating," he told me. "And the joint pain I see is not nearly as bad as nerve pain, which is a whole level above. But even with patients in pain,

I try to get my patients to just move. If I can get them to do something, even just get in a pool for a short amount of time and walk, they almost always come back and tell me that they feel better and have less pain."

Dan tries to keep his patients functional in the face of pain. What's interesting about Dan is that he's also an ex-Navy SEAL. During his training, he saw why some people quit.

"All you had to do was just not quit," Dan recalled. "That's all they were looking for, the people who wouldn't quit." During Dan's training to be a surgeon, his experience with SEAL training was incredibly beneficial. It had taught him resilience.

"When you realize you need to have your shit together to survive a night-time parachute jump, get onto a raft in 10-foot ocean swells, and then start the motor and get to land, you very quickly get your priorities straight. More than anything, no matter how bad the training got, no matter the situation, the idea was *never quit. Never ring the bell. Never give up.*"

Dan feels his experiences have helped him be a better surgeon, particularly when there is an unstable patient, or when things aren't going exactly as planned in the operating room. "You take a step back, get the priorities straight, and do your best under pressure...and you never quit on a patient."

This never-give-up attitude translates into better resilience with pain. Pain, in some ways, forces us to prioritize what is happening. If you find yourself lacking direction, pain will jolt you into action. The key is to maintain function as much as possible. Dan finds that keeping patients functional is a critical part of maintaining perspective on resilience. To some degree, function is always what we want to maintain in the face of chronic pain, even if we have to give a patient opiates to be functional. Zero pain is not the goal, but avoiding zero function is.

When great athletes meet in the sports arena, we often see how they mirror our lives. We are inspired. We take lessons to heart from sports that we can use in our own struggles. So many examples come to mind: Tiger Woods winning the U.S. Open in 2008 with an ACL tear. Michael Jordan scoring 38 points in the 1997 NBA finals with the flu. Eric Montross of UNC enduring a hard elbow and bloody cheek by Christian Laettner of Duke to prevail in the Tobacco Road matchup in February 1992.

Remembering Henry Beecher—strong emotions can block out pain—we appreciate our athletes even more when they are pushed into their pain zones in the spirit of competition and show good sportsmanship. We are proud to see them face their pain and rise above it, putting the team or the competition above their individual suffering.

In closing, I hope that this book has helped you understand pain better. The advantages of having pain in our lives outweigh the negative consequences of living without pain. Pain's guiding qualities cannot be ignored, and if monitored closely, can be a powerful instrument for growth and change. Is it time to change our perspective on chronic pain in the United States?

Sergeant Shane Savage fought in Iraq and was profiled in the *New York Times*. Savage was serving his fourth tour in

Iraq when he was severely injured by a roadside bomb. He was placed on opioids for chronic pain. He also struggled with the psychological trauma from the war. He even tried to commit suicide at one point. Then Savage came to a turning point, weaning himself off opioids and starting a program to help others with chronic pain do the same. Today he feels much more in control of his life.

Dr. Christopher Spevak, a physician at Walter Reed, says that "as we decrease the amount of opioids . . . healing and recovery has gotten much quicker." Walter Reed decreased the number of patients on chronic opioids from 80 percent to 10 percent from 2009 to 2014.

A patient came to see me with shooting pain down his leg. To my surprise, I found that his pain didn't go where it typically would have based on the atlas of the human body. The more I practice medicine, the more I discover that actual humans don't really follow the textbooks consistently, or at all for that matter. To some degree, the path pain takes, well, it's a lot like the path we each take in life—anything but a straight road.

In fact, when we think things are headed on a straight path somewhere, it is pain that often shocks us off that path until we can pull ourselves together and chart a new course. I would ask you to use the energy of pain to transform yourself and to help guide you on your path forward.

ACKNOWLEDGEMENTS

I WANT TO TAKE a moment to thank all of the wonderful people who helped me see this book through to completion. It wasn't easy to write a book while practicing full-time as a pain management physician. What I realized through this arduous process is that when you have a message to share with others, you quickly learn how to prioritize and just simply make it happen.

A special thanks to my wife, Naina, and my daughter, Ariyana, for their love and support, without which I would have long ago given up hope of completing this book. I am certain I crossed their pain thresholds and perhaps their pain tolerances a number of times while writing this book. I also want to thank all the folks (some names mentioned, some not) in this book who took time out of their busy schedules to speak to me about pain, and allowed me to see important points from other perspectives which helped me provide balance and texture to some of the concepts that I have conveyed.

I want to especially thank my fantastic editors, David Moldawer, Christina Verigan, and Laura Parker. I've never been a naturally gifted writer, but they helped me elevate my game to a level that I would not have achieved on my own. I jokingly said to them on several occasions that there is a reason I became a physician, not a writer. I also want to thank Rohit Bhargava for taking me on as a first-time author and for his help in publishing this book, as well as Marnie McMahon and all the wonderful folks at IdeaPress Publishing who helped shepherd this project from start to finish.

I want to also thank all the patients who took time to revisit some of their painful experiences while speaking to me about their struggles. I am certain it was not easy living through the original experience (nor the re-experience) of the pain when conveying thoughts, emotions, and feelings about their ordeals. You have helped me (and through me, the readers) see pain better and I am certain others will benefit from your painful experiences.

Most of all, I want to thank all the patients over the years who trusted me with their care and took the time to share their pain with me. Without this education, I would never have arrived where I am today regarding my understanding of pain.

FINAL THOUGHTS

PAIN IS BOTH OVERTREATED and undertreated. In the words of Dr. Tom Lee, there is simply no "getting it right" with pain. This is a harsh reality of the world we live in. Overtreatment leads to overdose deaths from opiate medications, and undertreatment leads to unnecessary suffering. We as pain management specialists have a special calling to be the final arbiters of the decision to treat and manage pain individually and to master a complex art and science. How do we navigate our route? Like Daedalus, flying with wings held together with wax just high enough above the sea but below the heat of the sun? We must not take the route of Icarus, who, enamored with his ability to fly, soared up to the sky, melting the wax in his wings, and then plunged to his death in the ocean. Like the wax that held together their wings, we must stick to safe and effective treatments to manage pain but also continue innovating to find new and better wings with which to fly with.

Dr. Lee also continues by saying that "greatness comes from starting with why." While we may wish for a life without pain, we know from CIP children that it is far better to have it than not. I hope that this book helps explain some of the why's of pain.

When we encounter pain, treat the underlying problem, and manage it when treatment is not a cure, and then find a healthy balance that does not rely too heavily on opiates. We must realize that zero pain is not the goal. Let us hope for a future that looks at better, more balanced treatments for chronic pain while we provide relief to those who are suffering...and let us meet the pain we face in life with resilience.

AUTHOR BIO

DR. SINGLA WAS BORN in New Jersey and grew up in North Carolina. After attending college at the University of North Carolina at Chapel Hill, he attended medical school at the University of North Carolina at Chapel Hill, where he graduated with Honors and spent additional time obtaining a Master's in Public Health, with a focus on Health Policy and Administration. Dr. Singla completed his Residency in Anesthesiology at Massachusetts General Hospital and subsequently completed an Interventional Pain Management Fellowship at Brigham and Women's Hospital, both affiliated with Harvard Medical School. During his residency, Dr. Singla also completed a fellowship at the Partners Institute for Health Policy, where he performed research in Patient Safety and other health policy research. Dr. Singla also served as the Chair of the Massachusetts Medical Society Resident and Fellow Section and was also a member of the Board of Directors (Committee on Publications) for the *New England Journal of Medicine*. Dr. Singla has had several appearances in media, including print, radio, internet, and television to address public health issues and most recently the topic of Pain Management. Dr. Singla has published several articles in medical literature and has performed research in Pain Medicine. He currently focuses his practice on minimally invasive options for the treatment of chronic pain. He continues to serve on the physician faculty at Harvard Medical School with the title of *Lecturer*.

REFERENCES BY CHAPTER

INTRODUCTION REFERENCES

Pizzo, P. A. and N. M. Clark (2012). "Alleviating suffering 101—pain relief in the United States." *N Engl J Med* 366(3): 197-199.

Institute of Medicine (U.S.). Committee on Advancing Pain Research Care and Education. (2011). *Relieving pain in America: a blueprint for transforming prevention, care, education, and research.* Washington, D.C.: National Academies Press.

CHAPTER 1 REFERENCES

Bourke, J. (2014). *The story of pain: from prayer to painkillers.* Oxford: Oxford University Press.

Franklin, B. (1916). *The autobiography and other writings.* New York: Henry Holt and Company. Retrieved from http://www.gutenberg.org/files/20203/20203-h/20203-h.htm (accessed October 25, 2016).

Hillenbrand, L. (2010). *Unbroken: a World War II story of survival, resilience, and redemption.* New York: Random House.

Kalanithi, P. (2016). *When breath becomes air.* New York: Penguin Random House.

McGonigal, K. (2015). *The upside of stress: why stress is good for you, and how to get good at it.* New York: Penguin.

Tolle, E. (2005). *A new earth: awakening to your life's purpose.* New York: Dutton/Penguin.

Woolf, C. J. (2010). "What is this thing called pain?" *J Clin Invest* 120(11): 3742-3744.

Yancey, P. and P.W. Brand (1997). *The gift of pain: why we hurt & what we can do about it.* Grand Rapids: Zondervan.

CHAPTER 2 REFERENCES

Caton, D. (1985). "The secularization of pain." *Anesthesiology* 62(4): 493-501.

Centers for Medicare & Medicaid Services (2016). "NHE Fact Sheet," CMS.gov website. Retrieved from https://www.cms.gov/research-statistics-data-and-systems/statistics-trends-and-reports/nationalhealthexpenddata/nhe-fact-sheet.html (accessed October 27, 2016).

Cuellar, J. M., P. M. Borges, et al. (2013). "Cytokine expression in the epidural space: a model of noncompressive disc herniation-induced inflammation." *Spine (Phila PA 1976)* 38(1): 17-23.

Descartes, R. and T. S. Hall (2003). *Treatise of man.* Amherst, N.Y.: Prometheus Books.

Dyck, P. J., J. F. Mellinger, et al. (1983). "Not 'indifference to pain' but varieties of hereditary sensory and autonomic neuropathy." *Brain* 106 (Pt 2): 373-390.

Haugeberg, G., S. Morton, et al. (2011). "Effect of intra-articular corticosteroid injections and inflammation on periarticular and generalised bone loss in early rheumatoid arthritis." *Ann Rheum Dis* 70(1): 184-187.

Hemlow, J. (1958). *The history of Fanny Burney.* Oxford: Clarendon Press.

Institute of Medicine (U.S.), Committee on Advancing Pain Research Care and Education (2011). *Relieving pain in America: a blueprint for transforming prevention, care, education, and research.* Washington, D.C.: National Academies Press.

Ji, R. R., Z. Z. Xu, et al. (2014). "Emerging targets in neuroinflammation-driven chronic pain." *Nat Rev Drug Discov* 13(7): 533-548.

Karthikeyan, M., T. Sreenivas, et al. (2013). "Congenital insensitivity to pain and anhydrosis: a report of two cases." *J Orthop Surg (Hong Kong)* 21(1): 125-128.

Keys, T. E. (1996). *The history of surgical anesthesia.* Park Ridge, Ill.: Wood Library, Museum of Anesthesiology.

Latremoliere, A. and C. J. Woolf (2009). "Central sensitization: a generator of pain hypersensitivity by central neural plasticity." *J Pain* 10(9): 895-926.

Lewis, C. S. (1962). *The problem of pain.* New York: Macmillan.

Moayedi, M. and K. D. Davis (2013). "Theories of pain: from specificity to gate control." *J Neurophysiol* 109(1): 5-12.

Perkins, B. (2005). "How does anesthesia work?" *Scientific American.* Retrieved from https://www.scientificamerican.com/article/how-does-anesthesia-work/ (accessed October 25, 2016).

Pizzo, P. A. and N. M. Clark (2012). "Alleviating suffering 101—pain relief in the United States." *N Engl J Med* 366(3): 197-199.

Riol-Blanco, L., J. Ordovas-Montanes, et al. (2014). "Nociceptive sensory neurons drive interleukin-23-mediated psoriasiform skin inflammation." *Nature* 510(7503): 157-161.

Talbot, S., S. L. Foster, et al. (2016). "Neuroimmunity: physiology and pathology." *Annu Rev Immunol* 34: 421-447.

Tolle, E. (2005). *A new earth: awakening to your life's purpose*. New York: Dutton/Penguin.

van den Bosch, G. E., M. G. Baartmans, et al. (2014). "Pain insensitivity syndrome misinterpreted as inflicted burns." *Pediatrics* 133(5): e1381-1387.

Wall, P. D. (2000). *Pain: the science of suffering*. New York: Columbia University Press.

Wheeler, D. W., M. C. Lee, et al. (2014). "Case Report: Neuropathic pain in a patient with congenital insensitivity to pain." *F1000Res* 3: 135.

Yancey, P. and P. W. Brand (1997). *The gift of pain: why we hurt & what we can do about it*. Grand Rapids: Zondervan.

CHAPTER 3 REFERENCES

Carr, L., M. Iacoboni, et al. (2003). "Neural mechanisms of empathy in humans: a relay from neural systems for imitation to limbic areas." *Proc Natl Acad Sci U S A* 100(9): 5497-5502.

Danziger, N. and J. C. Willer (2005). "Tension-type headache as the unique pain experience of a patient with congenital insensitivity to pain." *Pain* 117(3): 478-483.

Demeter, N., N. Josman, et al. (2015). "Who can benefit from virtual reality to reduce experimental pain? A crossover study in healthy subjects." *Eur J Pain* 19(10): 1467-1475.

Eisenberger, N. I. and M. D. Lieberman (2004). "Why rejection hurts: a common neural alarm system for physical and social pain." *Trends Cogn Sci* 8(7): 294-300.

Epictetus (1768). *All the works of Epictetus, which are now extant: consisting of his Discourses, preserved by Arrian, in four books, the Enchiridion, and fragments* (E. Carter, Trans.). London: J. and F. Rivington.

Fan, Y. T., C. Chen, et al. (2016). "The Neural Mechanisms of Social Learning from Fleeting Experience with Pain." *Front Behav Neurosci* 10: 11.

Foell, J., R. Bekrater-Bodmann, et al. (2014). "Mirror therapy for phantom limb pain: brain changes and the role of body representation." *Eur J Pain* 18(5): 729-739.

Goren, E. (2007). "Society's Use of the Hero Following a National Trauma." *Am J Psychoanal* 67: 37-52.

Green, W. (2015). "The World's Best Investors" (excerpt from *The Great Minds of Investing*), *Barron's*. Retrieved from http://www.barrons.com/articles/profiling-wall-streets-bright-lights-1432956817 (accessed October 29, 2016).

Guillory, J. E., J. T. Hancock, et al. (2015). "Text messaging reduces analgesic requirements during surgery." *Pain Med* 16(4): 667-672.

Guo, C., H. Deng, et al. (2015). "Effect of virtual reality distraction on pain among patients with hand injury undergoing dressing change." *J Clin Nurs* 24(1-2): 115-120.

International Association for the Study of Pain (2016). "IASP Taxonomy," IASP website. Retrieved from http://www.iasp-pain.org/Taxonomy (accessed October 28, 2016).

Jin, W., A. Choo, et al. (2016). "A Virtual Reality Game for Chronic Pain Management: A Randomized, Controlled Clinical Study." *Stud Health Technol Inform* 220: 154-160.

Kessler, R. C. and E. J. Bromet (2013). "The epidemiology of depression across cultures." *Annu Rev Public Health* 34: 119-138.

Kupfer, D. J., E. Frank, et al. (2012). "Major depressive disorder: new clinical, neurobiological, and treatment perspectives." *Lancet* 379(9820): 1045-1055.

la Cour, P. and M. Petersen (2015). "Effects of mindfulness meditation on chronic pain: a randomized controlled trial." *Pain Med* 16(4): 641-652.

Lee, J. H. (2016). "The Effects of Music on Pain: A Meta-Analysis." *J Music Ther* 53(4): 430-477.

Mee, S., B. G. Bunney, et al. (2006). "Psychological pain: a review of evidence." *J Psychiatr Res* 40(8): 680-690.

Osmond, H., R. Mullaly, et al. (1984). "The pain of depression compared with physical pain." *Practitioner* 228(1395): 849-853.

Porras, J. I., S. Emery, et al. (2007). *Success built to last: creating a life that matters.* Upper Saddle River, N.J.: Wharton School Publishing.

Shay, J. (1994). *Achilles in Vietnam: combat trauma and the undoing of character.* New York: Scribner.

Stollberger, C., J. Finsterer, et al. (2006). "Transient left ventricular dysfunction (tako-tsubo phenomenon): Findings and potential pathophysiological mechanisms." *Can J Cardiol* 22(12): 1063-1068.

Turner, J. A., M. L. Anderson, et al. (2016). "Mindfulness-based stress reduction and cognitive behavioral therapy for chronic low back pain: similar effects on mindfulness, catastrophizing, self-efficacy, and acceptance in a randomized controlled trial." *Pain* 157(11): 2434-2444.

Yager, J. (2015). "Addressing Patients' Psychic Pain." *Am J Psychiatry* 172(10): 939-943.

CHAPTER 4 REFERENCES

Allison, S. T. and G. R. Goethals (2011). *Heroes: what they do & why we need them.* New York: Oxford University Press.

Allison, S. T., and Goethals, G. R. (2017). "The Hero's Transformation." In S. T. Allison, et al (Eds.), *Handbook of heroism and heroic leadership.* New York: Routledge.

Beecher, H. K. (1946). "Pain in Men Wounded in Battle." *Ann Surg* 123(1): 96-105.

Beecher H. K. (1956). "Relationship of Significance of Wound to Pain Experienced." *JAMA* 161(17): 1609-1613.

Beecher H. K. (1960). "Control of Suffering in Severe Trauma: Usefulness of a Quantitative Approach." *JAMA* 173(5): 534-536.

Campbell, J., D. Kudler, et al. (2004). *Pathways to bliss: mythology and personal transformation*. Novato, CA: New World Library.

Campbell, J. (2008). *The hero with a thousand faces*. Novato, CA: New World Library.

Frankl, V. E. (2006). *Man's search for meaning*. Boston: Beacon Press.

Homer (1996). *The Odyssey* (R. Fagles, Trans.). New York: Viking.

Luttrell, M. and P. Robinson (2007). *Lone survivor: the eyewitness account of Operation Redwing and the lost heroes of SEAL Team 10*. New York: Little, Brown.

Mandela, N. (1994). *Long walk to freedom: the autobiography of Nelson Mandela*. Boston: Little, Brown.

McPeek B. (2007). "Pain and Subjective Responses." *Int Anesthesiol Clin* Fall; 45(4): 25-33.

Ramos, C and Leal, I. (2013). "Posttraumatic Growth in the Aftermath of Trauma: A Literature Review About Related Factors and Application Contexts." *Psychology, community & health* 2(1): 43–54.

Yancey, P. and P. W. Brand (1997). *The gift of pain: why we hurt & what we can do about it*. Grand Rapids: Zondervan.

Wikipedia (2016). "Franklin D. Roosevelt." Retreived from https://en.wikipedia.org/wiki/Franklin_D._Roosevelt (accessed October 29, 2016).

Wikipedia (2016). "Oprah Winfrey." Retreived from https:// en.wikipedia.org/wiki/Oprah_Winfrey (accessed October 29, 2016).

CHAPTER 5 REFERENCES

Califf, R. M., J. Woodcock, and S. Ostroff (2014). "A Proactive Response to Prescription Opioid Abuse." *N Engl J Med* 374(15): 1480-1485.

Centers for Disease Control (2016). "Injury Prevention & Control: Opioid Overdose." Retrieved from https://www.cdc.gov/drugoverdose/ (accessed October 15, 2016).

Centers for Disease Control (2016). "Injury Prevention & Control: Opioid Overdose, Understanding the Epidemic." Retrieved from https://www.cdc.gov/drugoverdose/epidemic/index.html (accessed October 15, 2016).

Chen, L., M. Sein, et al. (2014). "Clinical interpretation of opioid tolerance versus opioid-induced hyperalgesia." *J Opioid Manag* 10(6): 383-393.

Cheung C. W., Q. Qiu et al. (2014). "Chronic opioid therapy for chronic non-cancer pain: a review and comparison of treatment guidelines." *Pain Physician* Sep-Oct; 17(5): 401-414. Review.

Chou R, J. A. Turner, et al. (2015). "The effectiveness and risks of long-term opioid therapy for chronic pain: a systematic review for a National Institutes of Health Pathways to Prevention Workshop." *Ann Intern Med* Feb 17; 162(4): 276-286. Review.

Doverty, M., et al. (2001). "Hyperalgesic responses in methadone maintenance." *Pain* 90(1-2): 91-96.

Dowell D., T. M. Haegerich, and R. Chou (2016), "CDC Guideline for Prescribing Opioids for Chronic Pain—United States, 2016." *JAMA* 315(15): 1624-1645. Review.

Federal Drug Administration (2016). "Timeline of Selected FDA Activities & Significant Events Addressing Opioid Misuse & Abuse," Retrieved from http://www.fda.gov/downloads/Drugs/DrugSafety/InformationbyDrugClass/UCM332288.pdf (accessed October 30, 2016).

Fishman, S. M. (2005). "From balanced pain care to drug trafficking: the case of Dr. William Hurwitz and the DEA." *Pain Med* 6(2): 162-164.

Gusovsky, D. (2016). "Americans consume vast majority of the world's opioids," CNBC.com. Retrieved from http://www.cnbc.com/2016/04/27/americans-consume-almost-all-of-the-global-opioid-supply.html (accessed October 29, 2016).

Hoffman, J. (2016). "Patients in Pain, and a Doctor Who Must Limit Drugs," *New York Times*, March 16. Retrieved from http://www.nytimes.com/2016/03/17/health/er-pain-pills-opioids-addiction-doctors.html (accessed October 30, 2016).

Lee, T. H. (2016). "Zero Pain Is Not the Goal." *JAMA* 315(15): 1575-1577.

Silvergate, H. (2015). "When Treating Pain Brings a Criminal Indictment," *The Wall Street Journal*, June 12. Retrieved from http://www.wsj.com/articles/when-treating-pain-brings-a-criminal-indictment-1434148923 (accessed October 30, 2016).

Tierney, J. (2007). "Juggling Figures, and Justice, in a Doctor's Trial," *New York Times*, July 3, Retrieved from http://www.nytimes.com/2007/07/03/science/03tier.html (accessed October 30, 2016).

Volkow, N.D. and A.T. McLellan (2016). "Opioid Abuse in Chronic Pain—Misconceptions and Mitigation Strategies." *N Engl J Med* 374(13): 1253-1263.

Wikipedia (2016). "Purdue Pharma." Retrieved from https:// en.wikipedia.org/wiki/Purdue_Pharma (accessed October 30, 2016).

Wikipedia (2016). "William Hurwitz." Retrieved from https:// en.wikipedia.org/wiki/William_Hurwitz (accessed October 30, 2016).

Yancey, P. and P. W. Brand (1997). *The gift of pain: why we hurt & what we can do about it.* Grand Rapids: Zondervan.

CHAPTER 6 REFERENCES

Bowden, M. G., M. L. Woodbury, et al. (2013). "Promoting neuroplasticity and recovery after stroke: future directions for rehabilitation clinical trials." *Curr Opin Neurol* 26(1): 37-42.

Bruehl, S. (2015). "Complex regional pain syndrome." *BMJ* 351: h2730.

Ellis, A. and D. L. Bennett (2013). "Neuroinflammation and the generation of neuropathic pain." *Br J Anaesth* 111(1): 26-37.

Ferrari, L. F., O. Bogen, et al. (2014). "Second messengers mediating the expression of neuroplasticity in a model of chronic pain in the rat." *J Pain* 15(3): 312-320.

Grau, J. W., Y. J. Huang, et al. (2016). "When pain hurts: Nociceptive stimulation induces a state of maladaptive plasticity and impairs recovery after spinal cord injury." *J Neurotrauma*, Dec 20.

Groh, M. M. and J. Herrera (2009). "A comprehensive review of hip labral tears." *Curr Rev Musculoskelet Med* 2(2): 105-117.

Kim, S. H., S. S. Choi, et al. (2016). "Complex Regional Pain Syndrome Caused by Lumbar Herniated Intervertebral Disc Disease." *Pain Physician* 19(6): E901-904.

Perez, R. S., G. Kwakkel, et al. (2001). "Treatment of reflex sympathetic dystrophy (CRPS type 1): a research synthesis of 21 randomized clinical trials." *J Pain Symptom Manage* 21(6): 511-526.

Pizzo, P. A. (2013). "Lessons in pain relief—a personal postgraduate experience." *N Engl J Med* 369(12): 1092-1093.

Verrills, P., C. Sinclair, et al. (2016). "A review of spinal cord stimulation systems for chronic pain." *J Pain Res* 9: 481-492.

Wolfe, A. (2014). "Weekend Confidential: Ray Kurzweil," *The Wall Street Journal*, May 30. http://www.wsj.com/articles/ray-kurzweil-looks-into-the-future-1401490952 (accessed October 30, 2016).

Xu, J., J. Yang, et al. (2016). "Intravenous Therapies for Complex Regional Pain Syndrome: A Systematic Review." *Anesth Analg* 122(3): 843-856.

CHAPTER 7 REFERENCES

Abdi, S., et al. (2007). "Epidural steroids in the management of chronic spinal pain: a systematic review." *Pain Physician* 10(1): 185-212.

Andersson, G.B. (2014). "Epidural glucocorticoid injections in patients with lumbar spinal stenosis." *N Engl J Med* 371(1): 75-76.

Bicket, M. C., J. M. Horowitz, et al. (2015). "Epidural injections in prevention of surgery for spinal pain: systematic review and meta-analysis of randomized controlled trials." *Spine J* 15(2): 348-362.

Carragee, E. J. (2005). "Clinical practice. Persistent low back pain." *N Engl J Med* 352(18): 1891-1898.

Cuellar, J.M., et al. (2013). "Cytokine expression in the epidural space: a model of noncompressive disc herniation-induced inflammation." *Spine (Phila PA 1976)* 38(1): 17-23.

Devine, D. (2016). "Stephen Curry had platelet-rich plasma treatment on his right knee," Yahoo! Sports, May 4. Retrieved from http://sports.yahoo.com/blogs/nba-ball-dont-lie/stephen-curry-had-platelet-rich-plasma-treatment-on-his-right-knee-182950035.html (accessed October 30, 2016).

Deyo, R.A. (1986). "Early diagnostic evaluation of low back pain." *J Gen Intern Med* 1(5): 328-338.

Deyo, R.A., J. Rainville, and D.L. Kent (1992). "What can the history and physical examination tell us about low back pain?" *JAMA* 268(6): 760-765.

Deyo, R.A. and J.N. Weinstein (2001). "Low back pain." *N Engl J Med* 344(5): 363-370.

Friedly, J.L., et al. (2014). "A randomized trial of epidural glucocorticoid injections for spinal stenosis." *N Engl J Med* 371(1): 11-21.

Ghaly, R.F., et al. (2015). "Should routine MRI of the lumbar spine be required prior to lumbar epidural steroid injection for sciatica pain?" *Surg Neurol Int* 6: 48.

Groopman, J.E. (2007). *How doctors think*. Boston: Houghton Mifflin.

Iyer, S. and H. J. Kim (2016). "Cervical radiculopathy." *Curr Rev Musculoskelet Med* 9(3): 272-280.

Kawakami, M., et al. (2000). "Role of leukocytes in radicular pain secondary to herniated nucleus pulposus." *Clin Orthop Relat Res* (376): 268-277.

Kurzweil, R. (2012). *How to create a mind: the secret of human thought revealed*. New York: Viking.

Manolagas, S. C. (2013). "Steroids and osteoporosis: the quest for mechanisms." *J Clin Invest* 123(5): 1919-1921.

Paterno, J., et al. (2014). "Common Clinical and Correlative Pain Generators of the Cervical and Lumbosacral Spine." *MRI essentials for the spine specialist* (A. J. Khanna ed.), New York: Thieme.

Saal, J.S. (1995). "The role of inflammation in lumbar pain." *Spine (Phila PA 1976)*, 20(16): 1821-1827.

Sharon, H., et al. (2016). "Mindfulness meditation modulates pain through endogenous opioids." *Am J Med* 129(7): 755-758.

Singla, A. K., M. Stojanovic, et al. (2005). "Persistent low back pain." *N Engl J Med* 353(9): 956-957; author reply 956-957.

Smith, G.C. and J.P. Pell (2003). "Parachute use to prevent death and major trauma related to gravitational challenge: systematic review of randomised controlled trials." *BMJ* 327(7429): 1459-1461.

Stuart, R. (2013). "Does platelet-rich plasma treatment work?" *Men's Journal*, October 28. Retrieved from http://www.mensjournal. com/health-fitness/health/does-platelet-rich-plasma-treatment-work-20131028 (accessed October 30, 2016).

Wesner, M., T. Defreitas, et al. (2016). "A pilot study evaluating the effectiveness of platelet-rich plasma therapy for treating degenerative tendinopathies: a randomized control trial with synchronous observational cohort." *PLoS One* 11(2): e0147842.

Wolfe, A. (2014). "Weekend confidential: Ray Kurzweil," *The Wall Street Journal*, May 30. Retrieved from http://www.wsj.com/articles/ray-kurzweil-looks-into-the-future-1401490952 (accessed October 30, 2016).

Zeidan, F., et al. (2015). "Mindfulness meditation-based pain relief employs different neural mechanisms than placebo and sham mindfulness meditation-induced analgesia." *J Neurosci* 35(46): 15307-15325.

Zeidan, F., et al. (2016). "Mindfulness-meditation-based pain relief is not mediated by endogenous opioids." *J Neurosci* 36(11): 3391-3397.

CHAPTER 8 REFERENCES

Amstadter, A.B., J.M. Myers, and K.S. Kendler (2015). "Psychiatric resilience: longitudinal twin study." *Br J Psychiatry* 205(4): 275-280.

Beecher, H.K. (1946). "Pain in Men Wounded in Battle." *Ann Surg* 123(1): 96-105.

Csikszentmihalyi, M. (1990). *Flow: the psychology of optimal experience.* New York: Harper & Row.

Farman, G. P., D. Gore, et al. (2011). "Myosin head orientation: a structural determinant for the Frank-Starling relationship." *Am J Physiol Heart Circ Physiol* 300(6): H2155-2160.

Gladwell, M. (2013). *David and Goliath: underdogs, misfits, and the art of battling giants.* New York: Little, Brown.

Goldstein, C. L., N. B. Chutkan, et al. (2015). "Management of the Elderly With Vertebral Compression Fractures." *Neurosurgery* 77 Suppl 4: S33-45.

Greitens, E. (2016). *Resilience: hard-won wisdom for living a better life.* New York: Houghton Mifflin Harcourt.

Luttrell, M. and P. Robinson (2009). *Lone survivor: the eyewitness account of Operation Redwing and the lost heroes of SEAL Team 10.* New York: Little, Brown.

Mandela, N. (1994). *Long walk to freedom: the autobiography of Nelson Mandela.* Boston: Little, Brown.

Meier, B. (2014). "A Soldier's War on Pain," *New York Times,* May 10. Retrieved from http://www.nytimes.com/2014/05/11/business/a-soldiers-war-on-pain.html (accessed October 30, 2016).

Rutter, M. (2006). "Implications of resilience concepts for scientific understanding." *Ann N Y Acad Sci* 2006. 1094: 1-12.

Wikipedia (2016). "Starling Law." Retrieved from https://en.wikipedia.org/wiki/Frank%E2%80%93Starling_law (accessed October 30, 2016).

INDEX